DETOX
H A N D B O O K

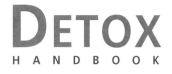

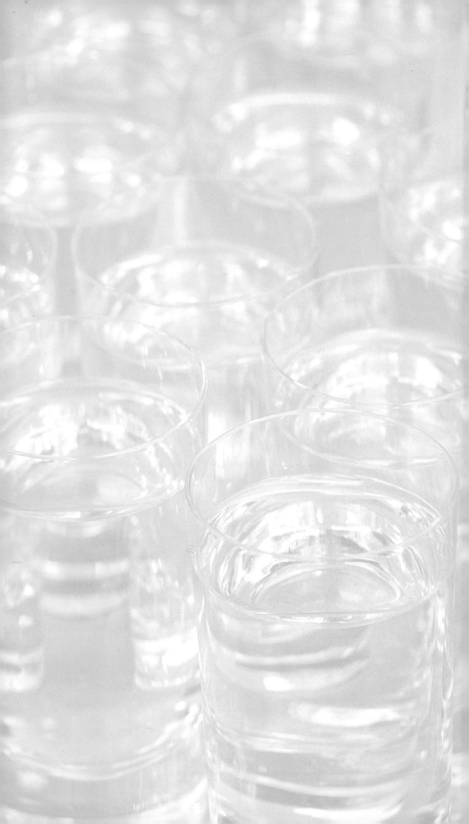

DETOX
HANDBOOK

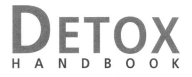

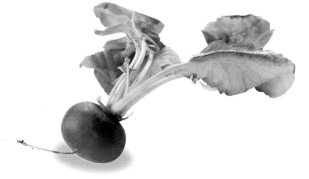

DR. JENNIFER HARPER
PHD MSc ND

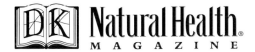
Natural Health® MAGAZINE

LONDON, NEW YORK, MUNICH,
MELBOURNE, DELHI

Natural Health magazine is the leading publicaton in the field of natural
self-care. For subscription information call 800-526-8440 or visit
www.naturalhealthmag.com. Natural Health® is a registered trademark
of Weider Publications, Inc.

In loving memory of my father

Project Editor **Janice Anderson**
Senior Art Editor **Margherita Gianni**
Senior Editor **Penny Warren**
US Editors **Jill Hamilton, Connie Novis**
Managing Editor **Stephanie Farrow**
Managing Art Editor **Mabel Chan**
Designers **Mark Cavanagh, Emma Rose, Axis Design Editions**
DTP Designer **Karen Constanti**
Production Manager **Joanna Bull**

First American Edition, 2002
2 4 6 8 10 9 7 5 3 1
Published in the United States by DK Publishing, Inc.
375 Hudson Street, New York, New York 10014
Copyright © 2002 Dorling Kindersley Limited, London
Text copyright © 2002 Dr. Jennifer Harper

Cataloging-in-publication data is available from the Library of Congress.
ISBN 0-7894-8441-2

Color reproduced by GRB, Italy
Printed and bound by South China Printing Co. Ltd., China

Consult a conventional medical practitioner if you have symptoms of illness while
detoxing or if you are on conventional medication and you intend to take dietary
supplements or have complementary treatments. If you are pregnant or breast-feeding,
only follow the nutritional advice for the level I detox program and do not use
reflexology and other spa techniques or take herbal medicines without professional
advice. See also the full list of cautions on page 9.

see our complete product line at
www.dk.com

CONTENTS

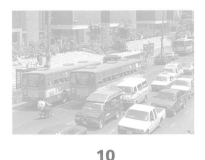
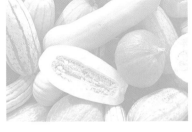
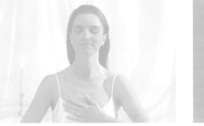
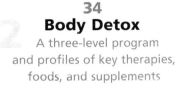

AUTHOR'S INTRODUCTION

Many natural health professionals consider detoxification to be the single most powerful tool in the prevention of disease. It is my desire to explain how detoxification works and to present a program that is safe and effective.

WHY DETOX?

Every day we are exposed to both external toxins (for example when we breathe in polluted air) and to internal toxins, which are created as a by-product of digestive and metabolic processes. If the body's immune system is strong and the organs of elimination (for example, the skin, kidneys, and colon) are functioning at optimum levels, the body is able to rid itself safely of these substances. However, for many different reasons the body may fail to eliminate toxins properly. If they are being taken in faster than the body can excrete them, a state of "toxicity" may occur. If this condition is left unchecked, it undermines one's health. In time it weakens organs of the body, and even contributes to a range of diseases including arthritis and irritable bowel syndrome (IBS).

MY DETOX PROGRAM

I have devised a holistic program to detox your body, mind, and spirit. It is divided into three levels, taking you from a gentle, nurturing detox at level 1 through to a deep, long-lasting cleanse in level III. The program is based on an unique combination of three elements: the wisdom of Eastern medicine, particularly that of Traditional Chinese Medicine (TCM), the tried-and-tested knowledge of natural medicine (naturopathy), and the latest research breakthroughs in Western medical science.

TCM AND DETOX

In TCM, illness is diagnosed and treated in a completely different way from how it is treated in Western medicine (*see pages 32–33*). Practitioners are trained to detect emotional and physical "imbalances" or "disharmonies," which can point toward a weakness in a particular organ or system. For example, to a TCM practitioner, frustration, anger, a green tinge to the face, and a sour taste in the mouth all point toward "disharmony in the liver."

By being able to observe such disharmonies, practitioners of TCM believe that they can detect signs of an imminent illness before the symptoms of the disorder actually emerge.

Throughout my program I talk about the symptoms of an overloaded, toxin-laden system as viewed in TCM because I believe that if you can become aware of these subtle indicators of toxicity in yourself, then you will understand better where your key problems lie.

I believe that the TCM approach to detoxing helps make my plan less austere and more in harmony with nature than other detoxification programs. People often experience a "healing crisis" (*see page 15*) while detoxing. With my program, any crisis you have is unlikely to be anywhere near as strong as it would be on a more conventional program, and so is less stressful for the body.

FUNCTIONAL MEDICINE AND DETOX

Practitioners of "functional medicine" aim to encourage all organs and systems of the body to function as well as possible. I have included new evidence and insight provided by functional medicine into the actual nature of detoxification pathways in the body. It is truly cutting-edge material that can lead us forward to a new level of understanding detoxification.

NEW APPROACH

There are very few similarities between my program and other detox plans you might have seen in newspapers and magazines.

My plan detoxes you slowly and gradually, unlike the usual style of detox programs. It works in tune with the body's elimination organs and does not encourage short fruit fasts, at the end of which you are likely to revert to your old bad habits. I believe that it is inappropriate to embark on a detox for a few days and then revert back to an unhealthy lifestyle. All that happens is that toxins are stirred up, only to become reembedded

A diet based on plenty of colorful vegetables, such as these peppers, nourishes body and mind.

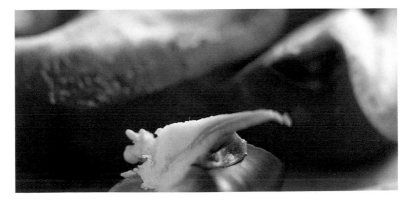

when the short plan is over. It is simply not feasible in a short space of time to expect to be able to deal with the mess that it has taken your body many years to get into. Instead, I want to encourage you to think of yourself as embarking on a journey, following a long-term program to a lifetime of good health.

A PLAN TO SUIT YOUR LIFE

Many people today have very high stress levels and are generally exhausted. My detox program has been designed with this in mind. It involves the minimum amount of side effects and stress and is there to be enjoyed rather than endured. Because life is so hectic, people are less inclined to comply with strict diet regimes, so adopting a manageable, gradual system is the best way forward.

MIND–BODY CONNECTION

Finding a balance between body and mind is fundamental to any self-healing program. This is why my book uses a variety of body, mind, and spirit therapies. My plan will give you a greater understanding of the connection between your health and well-being and your mind and spirit. The emotional and spiritual sections, among other things, will teach you to think about your attitudes to food and will give you the extra support and direction you need to

YOUR QUESTIONS ANSWERED

Here are some answers to questions I am often asked in connection with detoxing safely.

Q. Is fasting ever a good practice?
A. Because of the high levels of toxins from many sources present in the environment today, both inside and outside the home, I do not advise fasting. After undertaking a full detoxification program, it would be safe to follow a juice-only fast for up to seven days, but I am not an advocate of water-fasting.

Q. Can I follow the detox program in this book if I am pregnant?
A. I suggest that you follow the nutritional advice in level I (see pages 38–45), which is a sensible, supportive program that will help restore energy levels. However, you should discuss this with a healthcare professional first and ensure that when reducing certain foods that you substitute others wisely so that you get the full range of nutrients you need. You should avoid using herbs and spa techniques.

Q. Will I lose weight on this program?
A. It is likely that you will experience some degree of weight loss in the form of fluid loss. This is because the body retains water when the toxic load is high in an attempt to "dilute" the toxins.

Q. How often should I detox?
A. In TCM, the spring and the fall are the best times of the year to detoxify. You could follow levels I and II in the fall, which is the best time to cleanse the colon. Then follow the entire program from level I to level III in the spring.

CAUTIONS

You should not follow a detoxification program without getting professional advice first:

◆ if you are pregnant or are breast-feeding a baby. In particular, do not use spa techniques that involve essential oils or massaging reflex points and do not take herbal medicines without professional advice.

◆ before or soon after any major surgery when the body is weak

◆ if you are suffering from any long-term physical or mental illness

◆ if you are over 65 or under 18

stay motivated. You will intuitively develop your "spark within," which will help you to make potent and far-reaching changes for the better in your life.

DETOX AND YOUR DOCTOR

The information I give is not intended to replace conventional medical care, but should be used to complement the advice from your doctor. You should keep your doctor informed of how you are trying to help yourself and seek advice from a qualified practitioner if you have any queries. If you have any doubts regarding your state of health or already have a medical complaint, consult your doctor before starting this program.

COMMIT TO DETOX

This book is a wake-up call written with passion and compassion to encourage you to look hard at your present state of health and well-being and to decide how you can turn things around for

Investing time planning your detox program will pay rich dividends.

the better. It tells you all you need to know to undertake a fully beneficial detox program. If you want to know more, there's a list of books at the end of this book.

Your body has an innate desire to be well and to perform at an optimum level. If you cherish it instead of persisting with destructive practices, it will reward you with continued good health.

You should view this program in a positive light and look forward to giving yourself the love and respect you deserve – it's a chance to truly blossom and glow. *Angels fly because they take themselves lightly ...* don't get too bogged down with details. This detox time is meant to be exciting and fun.

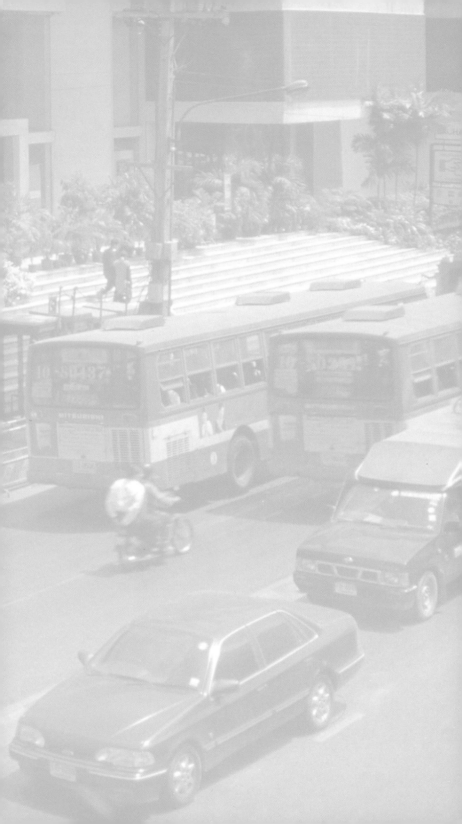

Why Detox?

Never before has mankind been so exposed to such a vast array of toxic compounds arising from pesticides, chemicals, inhalants, exhaust fumes, drugs, heavy metals, and radiation. Embarking on a detoxification program is the first step toward reducing the detrimental impact of these toxins on our health.

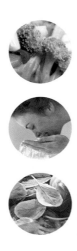

WHY DETOXIFICATION IS NECESSARY

If you have an average Western lifestyle and suffer from a range of minor ailments, it is highly likely that you need to detox. My programs reduce your "toxic load" and leave you with increased energy and zest for life.

THREATS TO HEALTH

Detoxification neutralizes toxins and removes them from the body by helping the elimination organs (skin, bowels, kidneys, liver, and lungs) to function efficiently. This process has never been so crucial: every day we face a barrage of toxic environmental compounds, which in time are thought to disrupt the body's ability to regulate key biological processes necessary for health, growth, and reproduction.

Current Western lifestyles add to the problem. Many people have raised stress levels and a diet that is high in sugar, fat, and processed foods and low in key nutrients. Such a lifestyle abuses the delicate working of the body and inhibits "detoxification pathways" – two phases of detoxification in the liver that neutralize and eliminate toxins.

Naturopaths believe that the widespread incidence of hormonal problems, fatigue, muscular aches, headaches, infections, debilitating viral illnesses, digestive problems, allergies, and even many forms of cancer all indicate that the "toxic load" is too high.

Too many toxins may weaken the body and the overuse and misuse of antibiotics reduce the body's ability to attack and destroy new strains of resistant bacteria and virulent viruses. In this way your system can become increasingly vulnerable and prone to a variety of debilitating infections.

The beneficial effects of a diet based on nutritious fresh foods, with the emphasis on vegetables and fruits, dairy products, and carbohydrates, cannot be overestimated.

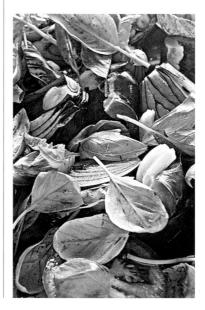

IMMUNE SYSTEM STRUGGLING TO COPE

An increased toxic load is thought to adversely affect the working of the immune system, which is programmed to defend the body from invasion by viruses and harmful bacteria. Food sensitivities and allergies are thought to be early signs that the body has become compromised in some way and that the immune and digestive systems have become weakened. Doctors may prescribe drugs for allergies, such as antihistamines to alleviate the acute allergic symptoms but these fail to address the root cause – the body's toxin overload.

DIGESTION AND TOXINS

Poor digestion, a sluggish colon, inadequate elimination of toxins through the digestive tract and the skin, and reduced liver and kidney function all contribute to increased levels of toxicity and impair the body's ability to function well.

In a poorly functioning digestive tract there can be increased growth of bacteria and yeasts, which ferment undigested food residues, turning them into reactive compounds. These are then reabsorbed by the body – a process known as "autointoxification." Finally, there are so-called "friendly" bacteria in the gut that aid digestion and health. Increased numbers of destructive bacteria and yeasts can overpower the friendly bacteria, thus further encouraging toxins to proliferate.

STRESS INCREASES TOXIC LOAD

Continuous stress adds to your toxic load. Research has found that high levels of stress hormones, such as epinephrine and cortisol, can shift "beneficial detox pathways" toward "harmful detox pathways," which encourage toxins such as free radicals to proliferate. This faulty detoxification can also cause high levels of stress hormones to accumulate in the blood. These are a major cause of health problems and may eventually lead to the development of serious degenerative diseases, such as heart disease and cancer.

We all lead ever more stressful lives; the need for effective detoxification of mind, body, and spirit has never been more vital.

THE BENEFITS OF A SUCCESSFUL DETOX

A carefully followed and successfully completed detoxification program can produce many dramatic results, including:

- increased energy
- improved sleep patterns
- decreased bloating and fluid retention
- reduced aches and pains
- improved mental clarity and memory
- a feeling of rejuvenation on all levels
- a sense of peace or calm

ANATOMY OF A CLEANSE

Like a team in a relay race, the "superficial" and then the "deep" eliminatory organs of the body work in a sequential order to remove toxins. My detox program works in harmony with the body for optimum results.

OUR MODERN WESTERN DIET

Our diet has changed greatly from that of our ancestors, who lived a very simple life in comparison with ours, eating unrefined fruits, nuts, vegetables, whole grains, roots, herbs, and other produce. This diet was rich in the essential nutrients, such as vitamins, minerals, amino acids, and enzymes required to maintain optimum health of both body and mind.

In the past hundred years or so we have turned to technology and chemistry to help provide food for the world's rapidly increasing population. This has resulted in the adulteration of many foods and the creation of the "Western" diet that is rich in processed and refined foods (starches and sugars), stimulants (caffeine), pasteurized dairy products, and high levels of saturated fats. If eaten to excess, these foods are thought to burden the liver and the immune system, eventually causing these organs to go into decline. We all need to return to a more natural diet, by way of a properly planned detoxification program.

LIVING NATURALLY

My detoxification plan is closely allied to two of the world's great natural health care systems, naturopathy and Traditional Chinese Medicine (TCM).

A belief in the healing power of nature is fundamental to naturopathy (*see page 26*), which believes disease results from the violation of "natural laws." The fundamental principle of naturopathy is to live in step with the constructive energies of nature to create a situation of harmony and balance within the body that allows healing to take place. Naturopathy follows commonsense rules, believing that for good health we need pure food and water, sunshine, fresh air, adequate rest and sleep, and the right amount of exercise. This is preventive medicine in its most efficient form.

TCM (*see pages 32–33*) believes that we should live in harmony with nature and that illness results when we transgress from living according to the laws of nature and fail to adapt to the natural changes of the environment and the seasons.

DETOXING SLOWLY

Detoxification has always been used in naturopathy to eliminate waste and revitalize the body. Popular cleanses today tend to focus on a weekend detox or a seven-day program based around a high raw fruit and vegetable intake, or fruit-only cleanses that have been adapted from a naturopathic regime.

While raw foods are very good cleansers, they are not always appropriate at the beginning of a cleansing plan. Unless you already consume large amounts of raw foods, changing from a Western diet to one of raw foods can swing your body into "shock cleansing."

On an all-raw food diet, especially one based on fruit, stored toxins are brought up from the "deep" organs, such as the liver, to the "superficial" organs of elimination – the skin, intestines, and lymphatic system. If these organs have not been prepared, considerable strain is put on them, triggering a "healing crisis," which is a cleansing reaction that occurs when toxic substances are expelled faster than the organs of elimination can remove them, leading to toxicity in the blood and lymph.

TCM practitioners say if a person is "deficient" or fatigued, stringent fasts or a raw food diet can lead to greater weakness. They believe the body must adapt gradually to new foods, the objective being to nourish and support the body while reducing dietary stressors.

Bearing these principles in mind, my plan begins slowly, strengthening the digestion in level 1, prior to allowing the superficial eliminatory organs to adapt to the cleansing program.

Cooked organic vegetables are kind to a stressed, toxin-laden system.

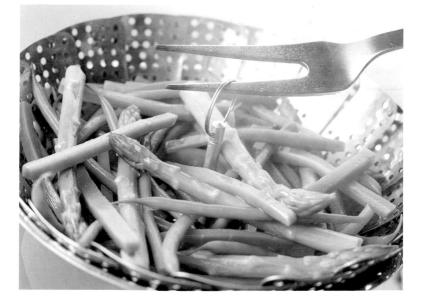

THE BODY'S ATTEMPTS TO STAY HEALTHY

The body has a natural urge to maintain homeostasis (that is, the situation in a healthy body when organs and systems continually adjust in order to maintain a perfect equilibrium or balance). Maintaining this state of perfect equilibrium – including eliminating toxins as necessary – is not easy. If the body is constantly pushed to the limits and is malnourished, at some stage it will become exhausted and no longer able to achieve homeostasis.

The ability to eliminate toxins differs from individual to individual. Specific nutritional requirements also differ considerably, depending on the individual's constitution and biochemical makeup. If you have an average Western lifestyle but have been blessed with a strong constitution, you may be symptom-free for a longer period than others, but if you are genetically weaker, toxins in your body may build up quickly and symptoms of ill health, both physical and mental, will soon appear.

NATURAL ORDER OF DETOX

The body is equipped with organs of elimination that all work together almost like a relay team, in a natural, sequential order. This balanced detoxification program works in harmony with the body through three levels. In level I the spleen and stomach enhance and support the digestion prior to the next leg (level II) which involves elimination. In this second leg, the lungs, colon, lymphatic system, and skin take the baton, and in the final stretch (level III) the kidneys and liver take over to complete the cycle of detoxification. The result is that toxins are released gradually and in a way that the body can manage.

Level I is a gentle program that supports the digestion. The aim of the level II program is to release toxins and fecal matter from the intestines and to ensure that the skin, lymphatic system, and lungs are working well so that they can expel additional toxins when the need arises during the final program (level III), which focuses on the liver and kidneys – the deep organs of elimination. (*For a detailed guide to the three levels, see pages 19–21.*)

In the fall it is a good idea to focus on seasonal produce, such as pumpkin and squashes, to cleanse the body in preparation for the winter season.

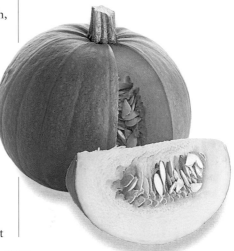

CLEANSING AND THE CHANGING SEASONS

The growth of plants mirrors the changing energy of the seasons. Some tubiferous plants grow underground in winter. In spring, other plants, such as spring greens, grow upward and outward above the ground. Likewise, the body's energy rises and moves from deep within during winter to the surface in spring.

According to TCM, the subtle energy (or *qi*) of foods nourish our own energy systems. There are seasons in nature when we should restore and nourish the body and there are periods when it is more appropriate to cleanse and detoxify (*see chart below*).

Ideally, we should try to synchronize our detox programs with the seasons and the body's cycles. If we understand this, we'll discover how to balance the extremes of each season and their effects on the body, as well as be able to make the most of the unique opportunities for growth that arise with each season.

NATURE AND THE BODY'S SEASONAL ENERGY

The best diet and detox program readily adapts to seasonal changes. Keep an open mind and be prepared to adapt your diet to suit the seasons and climate and to use produce that is grown locally.

Winter

Cleansing during the winter is not ideal. This is a time of hibernation, when replenishing energy stores and conserving and building the *qi* comes to the fore. A basic wholesome diet including cooked vegetables, grains like brown rice, and seaweed is ideal in these colder months. Try also warming spices including ginger, cinnamon, cloves, and cayenne. After this time of consolidation, you can begin to cleanse the body gently of the toxins that may have accumulated over this period of rest. Increasing your intake of vegetables and natural fiber ensures that the colon and superficial organs are able to clear wastes efficiently.

Spring

As you progress into spring, fresh green vegetables and herbs such as dandelion are abundant in nature. According to TCM, this is the time when the energy of the liver comes into power, so this is the most suitable time to focus on a deeper cleanse. Just as we traditionally "spring clean" our homes at this time of the year, so it is a good time to detoxify mind, body, and spirit.

Summer

Summer is the season when plants reach their optimum growth and your physical energy is at its strongest. You want to eat lighter, more cleansing foods to counteract the effect of heat. Summer is an essential time to build and restore energy levels to serve as energy reserves in the cooler months when energy is lower.

Late Summer and Fall

This is the time associated in TCM with the large intestine, lungs, and skin. It is a time to reflect on the past year and "let go" on all levels in preparation for the winter season, a time to retreat and consolidate. This is another good period in the year to cleanse the body, and colon in particular, and focus on seasonal produce, such as pumpkin and squashes, before the onset of winter.

NATUROPATHY AND DETOXIFICATION

Naturopaths say minor ailments such as colds, fevers, and boils and other skin problems should be seen in a positive light, because they are a sign that the body is trying to throw off an accumulation of toxins caused by an unhealthy lifestyle.

At the start of a cleanse, don't be surprised if your complexion becomes a bit dull or pimply. This is likely to happen because the skin is a superficial organ of detoxification through which toxins are eliminated from the deeper organs. Such outbreaks are usually shortlived and however irritating they may be, it is best not to treat them with medication. Naturopaths believe that attempting to suppress these natural reactions to detoxing with medicines has a detrimental effect on the body's innate intelligence and its natural healing power or vital force. They say that the danger of repeatedly suppressing minor ailments is that toxins are not expelled, the body's vital force is weakened, and the toxins are driven progressively deeper within the body. Toxins thus move closer to the core of your being and affect the deeper, more critical organs of the body. This means that complaints that do arise are likely to be more serious.

Drinking plenty of water helps the kidneys to flush out toxins from the system.

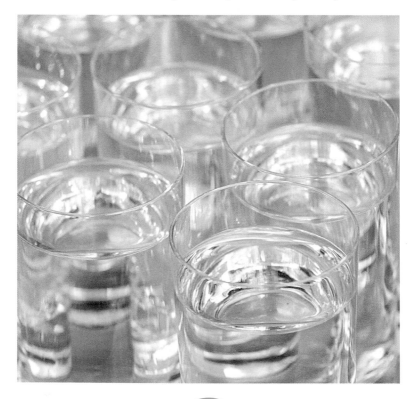

HOW TO USE THIS BOOK

Before you start detoxing, I suggest you read this book from start to finish so that you are familiar with the unique concepts it contains. Try to put out of your mind any detox plans you may have already encountered.

HOW THE BOOK WORKS

Compared with many recent books and articles on the subject, this book tackles detoxification from a very different perspective. It has a unique three-level approach that starts gently and becomes progressively more stringent.

Each level has three programs to detox body, mind, and spirit, as well as descriptions of key foods and therapies referred to in the programs. In each level, the body, mind, and spirit programs are designed to complement each other for optimum results.

I suggest you read about the three levels on the following pages and complete the questionnaire on pages 22–25. This will give you a clear picture of the main areas that need detoxifying and also provide a reference or base line prior to undertaking a program.

The questionnaire is invaluable for helping you to monitor your progress. Keep your original scores and do the questionnaire again when you feel you have completed a level, comparing your before and after scores.

WORKING THROUGH THE LEVELS

Irrespective of what you may already know about detoxing, you should start this detoxification program at level I and follow levels I to III in sequence. This is because the three-step program is rather like a pyramid in its structure, with level I forming the base. If the body is to be safely and effectively detoxified, each stage has to be thoroughly mastered before the next level is begun. Also, you should attempt simultaneously the body, mind, and spirit programs of each detox level, because you will only be ready to move onto the next level when there is harmony between body, mind, and spirit.

I suggest how many weeks each level should take, but there is no pressure to move to the next level within a specific time. It is far better that you move on only when you feel that the level at which you have been working has been successful. You should intuitively want to proceed to the next level and feel an excitement and enthusiasm for the journey and the changes ahead.

LEVEL I

This level is all about laying successful foundations for the detox program. If you do not detox properly at level I, your journey up through levels II and III will not be so successful.

The aims of level I are to nourish the body, strengthen digestion (which is allied to the Earth element in TCM), and to eliminate foods in the diet to which the body may be sensitive or intolerant.

I don't want to overload you (or discourage you) with instructions at this stage, so I have tried to keep the guidelines for the three level I programs simple (*For further details, see pages 40–45, 90–92, and 108–109*).

How Long to Spend at Level I

If you are new to detox and you eat a standard Western diet, you should stay at this level for at least four weeks. Do feel free to continue at this level for longer, and if you don't feel ready to move on, you can even stay here indefinitely.

If you already follow a diet similar to the one in level I (*see pages 40–41*) and you practice yoga and meditation regularly, you can reduce the time you spend at this level to seven days.

If your diet and lifestyle fall somewhere between the extremes of "good" and "bad" as described in this book, then two to four weeks at level I should be sufficient.

Getting Started

Level I involves eliminating certain foods from your diet (*see page 42*). If your life is very hectic, it may suit you to remove just one food group a week, rather than embarking on a full elimination diet immediately. Wheat would be a good food to eliminate first, substituting one or more of the recommended alternatives (*see page 39*). Easing yourself gently into a detox program in this way will minimize or avert a potential healing crisis.

If you are less rushed, you can substitute more than one foodstuff during the first week, but you should be aware that if you make dramatic dietary changes, you are more likely to have some kind of a reaction.

It is easy to assume that detox only takes place on a physical level. But you should not ignore the emotional and spiritual elements that are an essential part of this holistic program. Do ensure that you have assimilated the level I mind and spirit detox plans prior to moving onto level II.

Assessing Progress

Before you move onto the next level, repeat the level 1 questionnaire (*see page 23*). Has your score improved since you began? If so, you are now ready to experience level II.

LEVEL II

The aims of level II are to reduce exposure to substances that have the potential to weaken the immune system and to support the superficial organs of elimination (skin, intestines, lungs, and lymphatics). At this level you learn to let go physically, mentally, and spiritually (which is associated with the Metal element in TCM). Only when you feel that this

level has been reached and the body is working efficiently to eliminate superficial toxins and substances that cause inflammation, should you move onto level III.

I recommend that you spend four weeks at level II. As with level I, you should repeat the questionnaire afterward (*see page 24*) – your scores should be improved.

LEVEL III

It is essential that you carry out levels I and II thoroughly before you move on to level III. At this level, the body is being cleansed much more deeply, in a way that affects the kidneys and liver, the most important organs of detoxification. If you proceed too quickly to level III, toxins will be released faster than the insufficiently prepared kidneys and liver can deal with them.

For optimum results, you should allow four weeks for level III, although this can be reduced to two weeks if this is all that your schedule allows.

Essential Nutrients

The essence of level III, which is associated with the Wood element in Traditional Chinese Medicine (TCM), lies in eating foods that are rich in plant nutrients, essential fatty acids, and other beneficial substances, all of which have been validated by modern medical research as essential for health and detoxification.

These foods should be added to the nutritionally sound diet, rich in grains, light proteins, vegetables, legumes, nuts, and fruit, that you established at levels I and II (see pages 38–39). It is also important that you reduce your intake of refined, fried, and artificially sweetened foods.

After the level III program, the body should be robust enough to fight off the negative effects of stress and exposure to environmental toxins. You should be able to follow the diet element of level III as a preventive program for life.

Once you have finished, you should repeat the questionnaire (see page 25) to see how you have improved.

PLAN A PROGRAM THAT SUITS YOUR LIFESTYLE

As we have already seen in Anatomy of a Cleanse (see page 17), detoxing in harmony with nature serves to deepen and enhance the cleansing effect. It is important that you detox in tune with your body's own rhythms, carrying out the program at a pace which is comfortable for you. You should be gentle with yourself right through the process. You are a unique being and it is vital to find out what creates balance and harmony for you personally.

If you are new to this type of detox program, it is wise to begin over a weekend when you can have a few days at home to rest, just in case you need to. The first few days of each level are usually the hardest and the body may produce symptoms of toxicity such as headaches or tiredness as you withdraw from specific foods.

If you have a busy lifestyle, or one that takes you away from home, starting a program on a Monday or when you are staying in a hotel could leave you faced with unsuitable foods, coffee, and alcohol. It is better therefore to begin the program when you are at home and less tempted.

According to naturopathic theory, symptoms experienced before a detox may return for a short period of time as your body detoxifies. If this is the case, speak to a health professional who can advise you and, whenever possible, get plenty of rest and follow a healthy diet to support the body as it heals itself.

QUESTIONNAIRE

This three-part questionnaire can help you identify weaknesses in your health, whether physical or emotional. Completing it periodically throughout your detox program can help you assess progress.

PURPOSE OF QUESTIONNAIRE

According to Traditional Chinese Medicine (TCM), prior to illness, your body shows a variety of "imbalances." These can range from bowel disorders and headaches to more subtle signs such as an aversion to a color or taste.

THE RESULTS

When answering, try to be as honest as possible and go with your instinctive feeling, because this is likely to give the most accurate answer. Once you have filled in the questionnaire for a level (you will be starting at level I) add up your score. There are no good or bad results, but it is important to retain your score so that you can measure your progress after you have completed the program for that level. Ideally, your score will be lower once you have completed the detox program.

HOW TO SCORE

Quickly read the questions opposite and award yourself the following scores depending on the degree to which you suffer from the symptoms and emotions:

If You Suffer	Score
Severely	4
Moderately	3
Mildly	2
Infrequently	1
Never	0

Write down your score from your first answering of the questionnaire; you will need to compare it with later scores.

LEVEL I: DIGESTION AND THE EARTH ELEMENT

1	Poor digestion and assimilation of food		**11**	Inability to build strong muscle tone, weakness of the lower body
2	Slow metabolism and water retention		**12**	Lethargy and fatigue; a tired, "heavy" feeling in the body
3	Appetite imbalance, lack of appetite, or excessive appetite		**13**	Clammy, damp, cold skin and extremities
4	Abdominal distension and bloating after meals		**14**	Symptoms are aggravated by cold, damp, or humid conditions
5	Loose stools and gas		**15**	Discomfort under the left side of the rib cage (spleen and stomach)
6	Colic pains, acid reflux, and burping		**16**	Obsessional or compulsive feelings
7	Craving for sweet foods, the "chocoholic" syndrome		**17**	Easily worried, over-concerned, and over-whelmed by detail
8	Feel worse after eating cold foods or raw fruit and vegetables		**18**	Inability to nourish yourself, a lack of self-worth
9	Food sensitivities or allergies		**19**	Scattered feelings, poor concentration, not focused or centered
10	Fluctuations in energy levels due to blood glucose imbalances		**20**	A yellow tinge to the complexion

Total Score: [　　]

LEVEL II: ELIMINATION AND THE METAL ELEMENT

1 Bowel irregularities, such as constipation or diarrhea

11 Sinusitis or other nasal difficulties, including poor sense of smell

2 Strong odors from feces or gas

12 Hazy, muddled thinking

3 Bad breath, perspiration problems, and body odor

13 Dryness of the skin, psoriasis, eczema, and poor complexion

4 Poor lymph drainage, marked by body swelling; poor resistance to infection

14 Excessive mucus or, alternatively, dryness and lack of mucus

5 Lowered immunity, susceptibility to viral or bacterial infections

15 Craving for pungent, spicy foods

6 Coughing with or without phlegm, frequent throat infections

16 Pale skin color or a white hue

7 Fungal infections, including vaginal yeast infections, athlete's foot, and ringworm

17 Tightness in the chest or discomfort in the lower abdomen

8 History of antibiotics use or of use of the contraceptive pill

18 Inability to let go of the past, melancholy, nostalgia

9 Breathing difficulties, shortness of breath, asthma, emphysema

19 Grief, apathy, pessimism, and depression

10 Heightened sensitivity to environmental toxins

20 Inability to overcome negative feelings

Total Score:

LEVEL III: DETOXIFICATION AND THE WOOD ELEMENT

1 Nausea and vomiting

11 Symptoms including gout, hemorrhoids, and easy bruising

2 Headaches, migraines, and vertigo

12 Craving for sour foods, such as pickles and lemons

3 Difficulty digesting fatty foods

13 Frustration, irritability, anger, aggression, and shouting

4 Low tolerance to alcohol and caffeine

14 Jealousy and resentment

5 Premenstrual mood swings, tender breasts, irregular or painful periods

15 Emotional repression, unexpressed anger leading to depression

6 Stiffness, pain, or tight muscles in the shoulders and neck region

16 Poor organizational and planning skills, indecision

7 Tight ligaments and tendons, lack of flexibility, rigid attitude and body

17 Symptoms that are aggravated by wind and drafts

8 Sensitive eyes, poor eyesight, and spots in front of eyes (floaters)

18 Green tinge to the skin, especially around the face

9 Thin, weak, ridged, or split nails

19 Discomfort under the right side of the rib cage, near the liver

10 Pain under the right side of the rib cage near the liver and gallbladder

20 A metallic taste in the mouth

Total Score:

NATUROPATHY

Stimulates the body's self-healing powers ◆ Uses many

beneficial therapies ◆ Maintains health

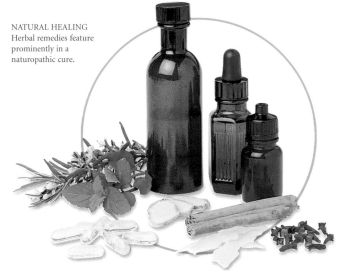

NATURAL HEALING
Herbal remedies feature
prominently in a
naturopathic cure.

KEY PRINCIPLES

Vis medicatrix naturae (the healing power of nature) is fundamental to naturopathy. It is thought that, given the right circumstances, the body can heal itself and stay in in a state of equilibrium called homeostasis, in which all body systems function properly.

Practitioners view disease as a sign that homeostasis is disturbed. They consider acute conditions, such as colds, fevers, and skin eruptions to be a form of healing crisis in which the body is endeavoring to eliminate toxins resulting from unhealthy living. Such healing crises are thought to be beneficial. Naturopaths believe that suppressing symptoms of acute diseases with drugs will result in toxins moving to a deeper level in the body. This will cause body tissues to degenerate and will contribute to the development of more serious diseases.

Instead of treating symptoms directly, naturopaths aim to strengthen the body's defenses so that it can detox and heal itself.

TREATMENT

A naturopath is an eclectic and will use a variety of therapies such as nutritional therapy, herbalism, massage, osteopathy, homeopathy, and relaxation techniques to help the healing process and encourage the body to return to its natural state of good health.

NATUROPATHY AND DETOX

Detoxification – the releasing of toxic matter to return the body to homeostasis – is fundamental to naturopathic practice.

◆ At level I, naturopathy works to enhance digestion and remove foods that stress the digestive tract and cause inflammation.

◆ At levels II and III, naturopathy aims to strengthen both the superficial and deep eliminatory organs so they can do their job.

NUTRITIONAL MEDICINE

Aims to remove allergenic and irritant foods ◆ Provides

optimum nutrition ◆ Supports the detox process

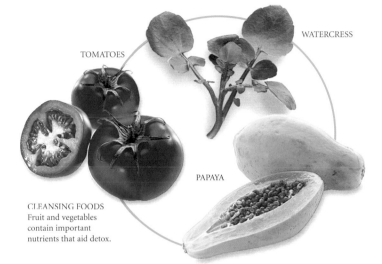

WATERCRESS

TOMATOES

PAPAYA

CLEANSING FOODS
Fruit and vegetables
contain important
nutrients that aid detox.

KEY PRINCIPLES

Nutritionists believe that the body needs nutrients from foods and supplements to enhance the function of weakened organs and tissues. Protein, vitamins, minerals, essential fatty acids, and a range of chemicals found in fruit and vegetables are just some of the nutrients needed for good health.

Many nutritional requirements are referred to as being "functional": when everything is working at an optimum level, there should be no need for more nutrients. When the body is placed under stress from other sources, such as emotions, infections, toxins, and radiation, or if illness already exists, the demand for nutrients is greatly increased. Nutrients previously not essential now become so if the depleted, stressed organ is to maintain function. Nutritional medicine aims to supply these increased requirements, while also identifying and removing the factors that caused the damage.

TREATMENT

Everyone is biochemically unique, and a nutritionist will design a tailor-made nutritional program, eliminating foods that stress the metabolism and increasing the amount of nutrients in the diet.

NUTRITIONAL
MEDICINE AND
DETOX

In a detox program, nutritional medicine can:
◆ At level I, remove potential allergenic foods.
◆ At level II, introduce gentle, cleansing foods to increase the removal of toxins.
◆ At level III, make use of phytonutrient-rich foods to enhance the detox process.

HERBAL MEDICINE

Potent form of natural medicine ◆ Improves digestion and

elimination ◆ Supports the body's self-healing powers

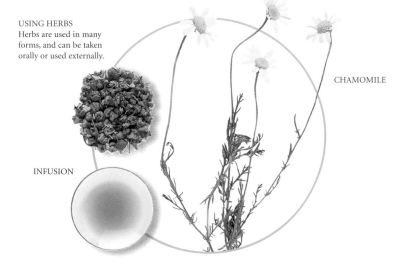

USING HERBS
Herbs are used in many
forms, and can be taken
orally or used externally.

CHAMOMILE

INFUSION

KEY PRINCIPLES

Herbs and spices have been used as medicines for centuries in many different cultures. In the West today, herbalism is one of the most widely practiced complementary therapies, its popularity helped by recent scientific research that validates ancient herbal wisdom.

Medical herbalists match herbs to symptoms and diseases and prescribe herbs to restore the body's self-healing powers. They say herbs have advantages over conventional drugs. Research has shown, for example, that some herbs are just as potent as many drugs derived from herbs but have fewer side effects. For example, white willow bark (*Salix*

alba) has the same pain-relieving properties as aspirin, which is derived from it. Unlike aspirin, it does not irritate the stomach lining.

Herbs contain many complex active ingredients that work together in synergy to make them a highly potent form of natural medicine.

TREATMENT

For best results, visit a medical herbalist who can prescribe a mix of herbs tailored to your condition. You can also buy dried herbs and herbal teabags, tinctures, fresh juices, capsules, and ointments. You should always buy herbs and herbal supplements from a reputable supplier.

● **CAUTION**
Always check: many herbs are contraindicated in pregnancy or under other specific circumstances.

HERBAL MEDICINE
AND DETOX

Herbs and spices are valuable in all three levels of the detox program:

◆ At level I, herbs and spices are suggested to aid the digestion.
◆ At level II, herbs help counteract fungal, bacterial, and viral infections, and speed toxin removal from the bowel.
◆ At level III, parsley, rosemary, and dandelion can aid deep detoxification.

AROMATHERAPY

Helps relieve digestive ailments ◆ Enhances the immune

system ◆ Relaxes and improves mood

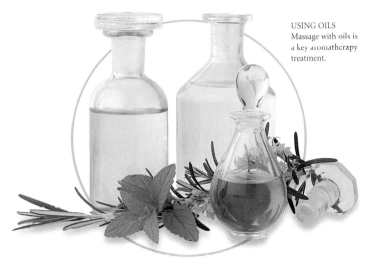

USING OILS
Massage with oils is
a key aromatherapy
treatment.

KEY PRINCIPLES

Aromatherapy, or phyto-therapy as it is also called, uses aromatic essential oils extracted from herbs, flowers, fruits, and trees. The oils are believed to penetrate the skin and be carried through the body via the circulatory and lymphatic systems.

Each oil is said to have an affinity with a system or organ in the body, as well as a specific therapeutic property, from detoxifying, stimulating, calming, or pain-relieving to antiviral and antibacterial.

The digestive and eliminatory systems are thought to respond well to aromatherapy, and the external application of oils may give relief from many ailments, including poor digestion, gas, and constipation.

TREATMENT

Aromatherapists usually recommend massaging with diluted essential oils, adding them to the bath, or using them in a steam inhalation. This allows droplets of oil to enter the bloodstream via the lungs or to help clear the respiratory system.

Essential oils are very potent and should not be taken internally or applied undiluted to the skin. As a general guide, mix 1 drop of essential oil with 1 tsp (5 ml) of a light vegetable carrier oil before use. If taking homeopathic remedies, be aware that strong oils such as tea tree, camphor, eucalyptus, and peppermint can antidote homeopathic remedies.

● **CAUTION**
Many oils are contra-indicated in pregnancy or other specific conditions. Always use oils diluted. Do not take internally.

AROMATHERAPY
AND DETOX

Using essential oils:
◆ At level I, oils help strengthen the digestive system.
◆ At level II, antifungal, antiviral, and immune-enhancing, oils are used.
◆ At level III, oils calm the liver. See Catalog of Spa Techniques (*pages 80–85*) for specific oils.

REFLEXOLOGY

Aims to disperse toxins ◆ Encourages the intestines and
liver to work well ◆ Believed to boost circulation

REFLEX POINTS
Pressing reflex points in
the feet has a beneficial
effect on the
corresponding part
of the body.

KEY PRINCIPLES

Reflexology is based on the principle that there is a relationship between the body's organs and systems and reflex points on the hands and feet.

The body is thought to be divided into ten vertical zones that relate to the ten fingers and toes. These zones run up the entire length of the body. The right side of the body corresponds with the right foot and the left side with the left foot, with "twin" organs, such as the kidneys and lungs, having reflex points on each foot.

In the 1930s, an American physiotherapist, Eunice Ingham, drew a map of the reflex points on the feet (*see page 121*).

Stimulating these points is thought to help eliminate waste products or "crystals" deposited in the feet. Circulation is improved, which allows healing to take place in the areas of the body that correspond to the points.

Reflexology is also believed to benefit the nervous system via the nerve endings in the feet.

TREATMENT

You should use your thumb to gently press on the reflexology point and "walk" along the whole reflex area, feeling for granular crystals. Small circular movements over any "crunchy" areas help to disperse the waste products. You should only work a reflex point

for 1–2 minutes and finish with a foot massage.

● **CAUTION**
Do not use reflexology in pregnancy and after a big meal or drinking alcohol.

REFLEXOLOGY
AND DETOX

Reflexology supports the body systems and organs worked on in each level.

◆ At level I, stimulating reflex zones aids the digestive system.
◆ At level II, the colon is supported.
◆ At level III, the focus is on the gallbladder, liver, and kidneys.

See Catalog of Spa Techniques (*pages 80–85*) for specific points to be worked.

ACUPRESSURE

Relieves "energy blockages" ◆ Helps to improve blood
and oxygen supply ◆ Aids relaxation

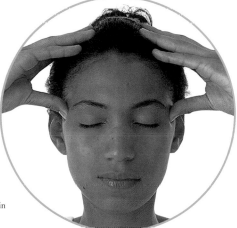

RELAXING
Pressure on specific
acupoints relieves pain
and reduces tension.

KEY PRINCIPLES

Acupressure is part of Traditional Chinese Medicine (*see pages 32–33*). It involves finger and thumb pressure to stimulate the same points that acupuncture treats.

The acupressure points are named and numbered according to the specific meridian (invisible energy channel) on which they lie. Practitioners of TCM believe that stimulating these points improves the flow of vital energy (*qi*) around the body through the meridians, which helps to relieve pain and many ailments.

From a Western point of view, acupressure is also beneficial because it relaxes the muscles, which helps to improve the blood and oxygen supply and release the buildup of chemicals such as lactic acid.

TREATMENT

Having located the acupoint, the aim is to stimulate the area that feels most uncomfortable to touch; this is a sign of congestion that needs to be released. Gently apply pressure with the pad of your thumb or fingertip, keeping the pressure light. Hold for approximately a minute. Alternatively, apply pressure intermittently by pressing on the point and then releasing. As your energy levels increase, you can use stronger pressure. Be sure to work acupoints equally on both sides of the body.

● **CAUTION**
Do not use acupressure in pregnancy and after a big meal or alcohol.

> ### ACUPRESSURE AND DETOX
>
> Acupressure detoxifies by decongesting meridian blockages.
>
> ◆ At level I, acupoints that increase energy levels are worked.
> ◆ At level II, acupoints stimulate the body's elimination processes.
> ◆ At level III, acupoints support the kidneys, liver, and gallbladder.
>
> See Catalog of Spa Techniques (*pages 80–85*) for specific acupoints used.

TRADITIONAL CHINESE MEDICINE

Encourages all systems to function at optimum level

◆ Aims to prevent health problems ◆ Boosts energy

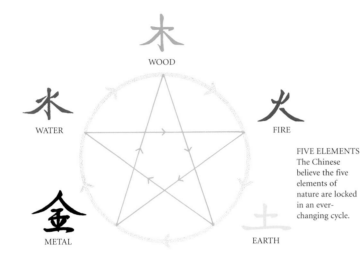

WOOD

WATER

FIRE

METAL

EARTH

FIVE ELEMENTS
The Chinese believe the five elements of nature are locked in an ever-changing cycle.

HEALING SYSTEM

With a 4,000-year-old history, Traditional Chinese Medicine (TCM) is one of the world's oldest forms of healing. In TCM, health is viewed as a complete state of well-being, which is a very different perspective to that of Western medicine, which defines health merely as "the absence of disease."

We can use the wisdom of TCM to isolate the best seasons to detoxify and to recharge energy levels. In addition, each of the detox levels in my program is associated with one of the five elements (*see right*).

KEY PRINCIPLES

Like naturopathy, TCM is based on the belief that humanity is part of the natural environment. It is thought that true health can only be achieved when we live in harmony with the environment and seasons.

Fundmental to TCM are the concepts of *qi*, *yin*, and *yang* and the five elements.

Yin and yang These are two opposing yet inseparable elements that coexist in everything. *Yang* is light, active, dynamic, and energetic, while *yin* is dark, cool, and passive. A balance of the two is needed for health.

Qi (Energy) is the invisible vital force or energy that the Chinese believe

TCM AND DETOX

Each level of the detox program relates to one of the five elements.

◆ Level I is connected to the Earth element, and aims to improve digestion and energy.

◆ Level II relates to Metal and "letting go" in mind, body, and spirit.

◆ Level III is associated with Wood and the cleansing of the liver and kidneys.

is present in all things. It nourishes and protects body, mind and spirit and its smooth flow is considered essential for good health.

Qi is carried around the body in channels (or meridians: see page 31) on which lie a network of 365 acupoints.

The Five Elements From their observation of nature's ever-changing cycles, the Chinese developed the theory of the five elements. This relates the five elements (Wood, Fire, Earth, Metal, and Water) to the different seasons and to the organs of the body, as well as to temperatures, colors, and tastes, all of which have relevance for our health and well-being. The table below sets out in detail the complex relationships between the five elements, nature, and parts of the body.

TREATMENT

TCM combines diet, exercise (such as t'ai chi and qigong), Chinese herbal medicines, and acupuncture in a unique therapeutic program to bring the body and mind back to a state of optimum health.

Practitioners of TCM aim to detect imbalances in the flow of qi and also to detect imbalances in the organs of the body before more serious symptoms can develop.

They use oils, herbs, and foods to balance yin and yang in the body. They also treat patients with acupuncture and acupressure to redirect and circulate the flow of qi to organs and to reestablish harmony in the body.

FIVE ELEMENTS TABLE

	Wood	Fire	Earth	Metal	Water
Direction	East	South	Center	West	North
Color	Green	Red	Yellow	White	Blue/black
Climate	Windy	Hot	Damp	Dry	Cold
Season	Spring	Summer	Late Summer	Fall	Winter
Yin Organ	Liver	Heart	Spleen	Lungs	Kidneys
Yin Time	1am–3am	11am–1pm	9am–11am	3am–5am	5pm–7pm
Yang Organ	Gallbladder	Small intestine	Stomach	Large intestine	Bladder
Yang Time	11pm–1am	1pm–3pm	7am–9am	5am–7am	3pm–5pm
Stage	Birth	Growth	Transformation	Absorption	Storage
Number	8	7	5	9	6
Planet	Jupiter	Mars	Saturn	Venus	Mercury
Spirit	Hun	Shen	Yi	P'o	Zhi
Parts of the Body	Ligaments/Tendons	Blood vessels	Muscles/Flesh	Skin	Bones/Marrow
Sound of Voice	Shouting	Laughter	Singing	Weeping	Moaning
Emotion	Anger	Joy	Worry/Sympathy	Grief	Fear
Taste	Sour	Bitter	Sweet	Spicy	Salty
Odor	Rancid	Burnt	Fragrant	Pungent	Putrid
Sensory Organ	Eyes	Tongue	Mouth	Nose	Ears
Reflector	Nails	Complexion	Lips	Body hair	Head hair
Secretion	Tears	Respiration	Saliva	Nasal discharge	Sputum

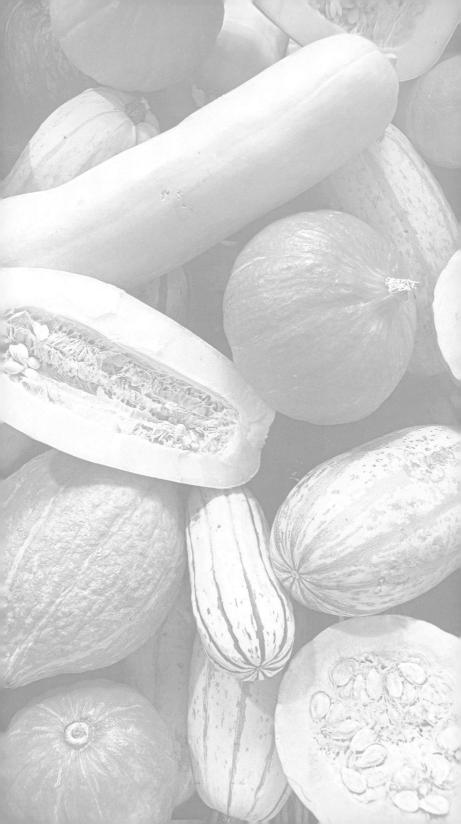

Body Detox

This three-level body detox program is rather like a pyramid. Its base is level I, where the program's foundations are firmly established. In level II, the focus is on reducing exposure to toxic substances and supporting the superficial organs of elimination. Level III, the pinnacle of the program, cleanses the body very deeply.

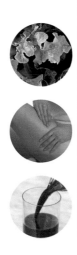

BODY DETOX EXPLAINED

The greater the array of stresses and numbers of toxins that penetrate the body, the deeper detoxification must go. The three-level program works in harmony with the body to restore balance and health.

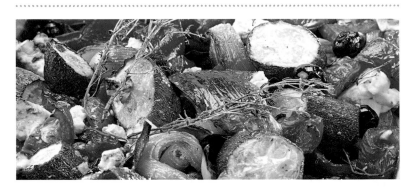

LEVEL I

This level in the body detoxification program has two main aims:

- To support the digestive system so that it can assimilate food efficiently.
- To reduce exposure to reactive compounds, such as food allergens.

Practitioners of nutritional medicine believe poor digestion and food intolerances are linked in a vicious circle. They say poor digestion is a precursor of food intolerances, which in turn go on to create problems with the body's ability to absorb nutrients.

Approximately half of the body's immune cells, whose job is to intercept and destroy harmful substances, are located in the gut. If digestive function is poor and food intolerances remain

A diet rich in sustaining cooked vegetables nourishes the body at level I in preparation for the detoxification program ahead.

uncorrected, this can lead to a breakdown in the integrity of the gut wall, thus contributing to food insensitivities.

In Traditional Chinese Medicine (TCM), the Earth element is considered to be connected to digestion. Practitioners believe food intolerances arise because the spleen and the stomach, the organs associated with the Earth element, are weakened.

Furthermore, practitioners of both medical traditions agree that, if you are nutritionally deficient or suffering from fatigue and are generally stressed, you must follow a properly planned nourishing diet before you start detoxifying. This will help your body recuperate and heal. Once strength is regained, the time is right to begin gently detoxifying the body.

LEVEL II

The level II program has three main aims:

- Reducing the body's exposure to "external" toxic substances.
- Releasing toxins held in the bowel.
- Improving and repairing intestinal function prior to the release of larger amounts of toxins in level III.

At this level, the program concentrates on the superficial organs of elimination. These organs – the skin, bowel, lungs, and lymphatics – correspond to the Metal element in TCM. Supporting these organs enables the body to let go of toxins stored in the superficial levels. It also strengthens immunity and increases resistance to infections.

REDUCE EXPOSURE TO TOXINS

It is essential that level II should be followed fully so that the body is cleared of both external toxins, such as pollutant chemicals, and toxins in the bowel (colon). Western functional medicine has identified two detoxification pathways, called phase I and phase II (see page 54). A toxic colon creates an imbalance between the phases and places stress on the detoxification pathways. The liver and kidneys, trying to detoxify compounds, are unable to cope with an extra toxic load coming from the colon. For this reason it is important to detoxify the colon properly in level II before moving on to detoxifying the liver and kidneys in level III.

IMPROVING INTESTINAL FUNCTION AND IMMUNITY

Louis Pasteur said, "le terrain est tout," meaning that the condition of the body determines whether harmful microorganisms will flourish or not. Poor digestion can encourage disease-producing bacteria and yeasts to multiply, which results in the production of harmful by-products, which inflame the gut lining. This may lead to intestinal permeability, which can cause bowel contents to leak into the body, a condition known as leaky gut syndrome. Therefore it is crucial to strengthen the gut to prevent the increase of harmful microorganisms.

LEVEL III

At level III, the program aims to:

- Support the liver and other deep organs of elimination.

The focus of level III is to detoxify the liver and kidneys. The liver is a powerful organ of detoxification and regeneration. It is also an essential part of the digestive process, producing nature's laxative, bile, which also helps with the digestion and absorption of fats. In TCM, the liver comes under the auspices of the Wood element and is believed to help filter the blood and detoxify the body. The kidneys remove toxins from the liver and eliminate body wastes.

PLANNING A DIETARY DETOX PROGRAM

Your detox diet will to some extent be an individual matter. Your meals will depend on your lifestyle, weight, fitness, and other factors. In addition to following the guidelines on these pages, you should also take note of the dietary advice within each level of the detoxification program. Avoid the asterisked foods at level II if you suffer from fungal infections.

BREAKFAST

On rising, drink a glass of hot water, with the juice of half a lemon if liked. Choose breakfast from the following:

◆ Millet or oatmeal (ideally organic) porridge. Use apple juice*, filtered water, or milk substitute to moisten.

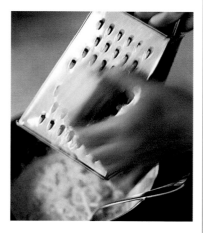

◆ Granola. To make, soak two tablespoons of oats overnight in water. Rinse in the morning and add apple juice*, a grated apple*, and a tablespoon of live yogurt.

◆ Add to the porridge or granola two tablespoons of soaked linseed,

sesame, pumpkin, or sunflower seeds (ideally semisprouted to increase nutritional value).

◆ Goat's or sheep's milk live yogurt with seeds sprinkled on top and some fresh enzyme-rich fruit such as papaya*, pineapple*, or berries*, grated apple*, or pear*. Or, blend these ingredients together to make a fruit-yogurt smoothie*.

◆ Two eggs, boiled or poached, with wheat-free bread or rice cakes, oat cakes, or similar.

MIDMORNING AND MIDAFTERNOON

Snacks at these times could be:

◆ Rice cakes or oat cakes with cashew or almond nut butter, eaten with half a banana*.

◆ A handful of mixed seeds with a few chopped nuts.

◆ Chunks of fresh fruit* or a fruit smoothie*.

◆ Glass of fresh vegetable juice, such as carrot, celery, or beet, with ginger or suggested fruits* added.

◆ Half an avocado.

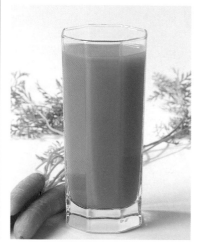

DRINKS

◆ Herbal tea, green tea, or coffee substitute with one of the cow's milk substitutes (*see list, right*).

LUNCH AND DINNER

For these main meals, there is a wide choice:

◆ Oily fish or organic poultry with plenty of vegetables.

◆ A vegetarian combination based around tofu, legumes, and grains (quinoa, millet, amaranth, or rice) with a few nuts (almonds, cashews, and hazelnuts), or seeds added. Brazil nuts are especially good at level III because of their high selenium content. Ideally, take nuts from their shells just before you eat them since they lose nutrients quickly once they are shelled.

◆ Homemade vegetable soup or vegetable stew, sprinkled with a few seeds, eaten with rice cakes.

◆ Brown rice or other grain with stir-fried or steamed vegetables. Choose colorful vegetables rich in plant nutrients, such as tomatoes, broccoli, carrots, peppers, onions, garlic, and dark-green leafy vegetables. Use boiling water or a small amount of olive oil to stir-fry.

◆ Baked sweet potatoes or roasted vegetables and an occasional baked potato (as long as you don't have arthritis).

◆ Sushi meals.

◆ A small salad of bitter greens can accompany any of the above dishes. Use a fresh dressing made with flax oil. Increase the amount of salad in level III to stimulate liver function.

◆ Desserts in summer can have enzyme-rich fruit* such as pineapple, or berries* with live yogurt. In the colder months, fruit* baked with warming spices, for example apple with cinnamon, is comforting.

A SIMPLE SUBSTITUTION LIST

You should not be daunted by the prospect of giving up certain familiar foods. There is a wide range of alternatives.

Wheat and rye products

Replace with rice, quinoa, millet, sago, amaranth, gram flour (used in popadoms), buckwheat, arrowroot, wheat-free pasta, soba and rice noodles, corn tortillas.

Cow's milk and products

Replace with rice milk, almond milk, oat milk, goat or sheep's milk, soy milk, mozzarella (made with buffalo milk).

Coffee and tea

Replace with chicory or dandelion-root coffee (although this may contain lactose and not therefore be dairy-free), herbal, or green tea.

Salt

Replace with seaweed and herbal salt substitutes. Use fresh herbs and spices instead of salt to give bland foods flavor.

Sugar

Replace with small quantities of carob, pure organic honey*, dates*, and maple* syrup.

NOTE Some of the foods on these pages (including the list above) are asterisked (*). You should avoid these foods at level II if you suffer from fungal infections.

PROGRAM FOR LEVEL I

The first level in the body detoxification program strengthens and supports digestion so that it can assimilate nutrients more efficiently. It also involves avoiding foods such as wheat and dairy products.

AIMS OF THE PROGRAM

Nutritionists believe good health depends on the digestive system working efficiently. Poor digestion and food intolerances are linked, creating a vicious circle. If your digestion is poor, you are more likely to have a food intolerance, which in turn can interfere with the absorption of nutrients. In time, this might lead to irritable bowel syndrome and other disorders. This level teaches you how to detect and avoid trigger foods, features nourishing foods rich in enzymes that improve the digestion, such as blueberries, pineapples, and beansprouts, and includes techniques and herbs to support and nourish the body.

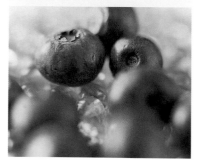

Your Program

- ◆ Follow the dietary guidelines and cut out unhelpful foods.
- ◆ Base meals around key herbs and foods (*see pages 59–73*).
- ◆ Tackle food intolerances (*see page 43*).
- ◆ Skin brush for 10 minutes every day. Then press the key acupoints (*see pages 80–81*).
- ◆ Do the stretching exercise every day (*see page 117*) and make time to rest in the day if you feel tired.
- ◆ For advice on how long to spend at level I see page 20.

Dietary Guidelines

Follow these guidelines.

- ◆ Drink at least eight glasses of pure mineral or filtered water every day to prevent dehydration and flush toxins out of the system. It is a good idea to mix water with saliva in the mouth so that it is, in a sense, digested. In TCM, cold water is said to weaken the digestion, so drink it at room temperature. Coffee substitutes and herbal teas such as peppermint or nettle can be drunk, but without cow's milk or sugar.

◆ Eat plenty of lightly steamed vegetables, stir-fries, and vegetable soups (*see box*, right, for a list of particularly beneficial vegetables). When stir-frying, avoid using oil, since fats change chemically when heated to high temperatures, becoming high in saturated fatty acids. Instead, use a little boiling water to start sweating garlic, onions, and ginger; when these have released some moisture, add the main vegetables.

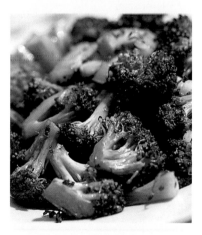

◆ Eat raw fruits in moderation in level I because they are potent cleansers. Pears are suitable because they are the least allergenic fruit and are also rich in insoluble fiber, which speeds up the passage of food through the bowel. Pineapple (which contains lots of enzymes) and antioxidant-rich berries are also good choices. Fruit is considered "cool and

damp" in TCM, so redress the balance with herbal teas made with warming spices such as ginger.

◆ Eat small quantities of good quality, lean organic protein each day to provide the body with amino acids. In TCM, protein (in small quantities) is viewed as beneficial, aiding energy levels and digestion. Eggs, poultry, oily fish (from unpolluted waters), and soy (as long as you are not soy-intolerant) are all good choices.

◆ Use cold-pressed virgin olive oil and flax, pumpkin seed, and walnut oils, which provide healthy essential fatty acids. Use them in fresh salad dressings.

◆ Choose whole foods and organic produce instead of ready-made meals and convenience foods.

Good and Bad Vegetables for Level I

Eat plenty of the following vegetables, which in TCM are believed to support the spleen and stomach:

◆ sweet potatoes

◆ potatoes (in small quantities)

◆ squashes, such as pumpkins

◆ parsnips, potatoes, carrots, and other root vegetables

Avoid the following, which are too powerful at this stage:

◆ raw vegetables (except sprouted seeds)

◆ onions and leeks, except in small amounts (for their quercetin content)

Natural Ways to Strengthen the Digestion

The body produces enzymes to digest and assimilate food. Some scientists think that the body has not yet made the necessary enzymes to cope with processed foods full of chemicals and preservatives. If the digestive system becomes weak through an inappropriate diet or stress, the levels of acid in the stomach can be reduced, impairing digestion still further, opening

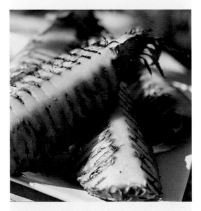

the door to various problems. To avoid this, you should:

◆ eat enzyme-rich foods such as pineapple and sprouted foods
◆ ensure that your diet is as natural and "whole" as possible
◆ drink ginger tea regularly before a meal and do not drink water while eating since this dilutes the enzymes
◆ avoid eating on the run since this does not give the stomach sufficient time to digest food
◆ take a digestive enzyme supplement (*see page 74*).

Foods to Avoid

You should cut back your intake of or preferably avoid the following altogether during level I detox. See page 39 for substitute foods.

◆ **Tea, coffee, chocolate, and other caffeinated drinks** These inhibit the absorption of vitamins and minerals and lead to dehydration. At least cut your intake to two cups a day and use organic varieties.

◆ **Alcohol** Drink no more than one glass a day of an organic red wine (and then only provided you aren't sensitive to tannins in red wine).

◆ **Fatty, fried foods, processed meats** Grill foods and follow the boiling water method of cooking stir-fries (*see page 40*).

◆ **Convenience foods, products containing sugar, and genetically modified or irradiated ingredients** Eat whole foods and organic produce instead.

◆ **Wheat and rye** These are onsidered to be "acidic." Wheat bran cereals can also scratch the lining of the colon. Instead, choose whole-grain oats and whole brown rice, which contains a high proportion of water.

◆ **Citrus fruits** such as oranges. These are considered to be "aggressive" cleansers, and if your liver is not as strong as it should be, it may experience difficulty in breaking down the fruit acids.

◆ **Dairy products** Milk increases the production of mucus in the body, so is not beneficial when considering a cleanse. See page 39 for alternatives.

What Is a Food Intolerance?

It is thought that over time the body can become intolerant of certain foods, failing to digest them properly. This can give rise to symptoms such as headaches, fatigue, and depression. Food cravings or symptoms such as headaches after withdrawing a food from the diet can be signs that you are intolerant of the food. Culprits can include ordinary foods such as milk, citrus fruits, and wheat. It is thought, for example, that many people lack sufficient quantities of lactase, the enzyme required to digest lactose, the main sugar in milk, and therefore cannot

Culprit Foods

The most common culprit foods:

- wheat
- cow's milk and dairy foods
- soy
- citrus fruits
- coffee and other caffeinated drinks
- tea (because of their tannins)
- certain nuts, especially peanuts

efficiently digest dairy products. Identifying the foods that are causing intolerances can be a problem because there is often a time lag of hours or even days between eating the food and experiencing adverse symptoms. Furthermore, sometimes more than one food can be involved.

TACKLING A FOOD INTOLERANCE

- Turn detective and try to isolate and determine what may be weakening your body. Keep a diary for about two weeks, noting everything you eat and how you feel.

- Choose at least one of the main food groups, such as wheat or dairy, and eliminate it from your diet for at least two weeks, but preferably four weeks. Be careful to eat the suggested substitute foods (*see page 39*) to ensure that no nutritional deficiencies occur. Eliminating foods temporarily gives your digestive system and immune system a chance to heal.

TAKE CARE

Remember, particularly if your schedule is hectic, that coming off a potential allergen can cause withdrawal symptoms such as fatigue and headaches, so you may need to rest and recuperate. If you begin to crave the food and have withdrawal symptoms, you should still abstain from the food in order to rest your digestive system.

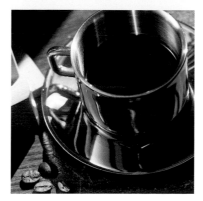

What Is Food-combining?

Food-combining is a useful regime that is employed to support digestion, because when foods are combined correctly they can be broken down more efficiently by the digestive system.

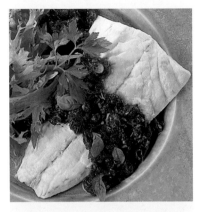

The principle is simple: do not eat concentrated starches (rice, pasta, potatoes, bread) and concentrated proteins (eggs, meat, fish) at the same meal. If your meal is mainly carbohydrate (for example, a baked potato), then eat other vegetables, including starchy ones such as parsnips with it. If you want to have fish, then you should not eat potatoes or starchy vegetables; instead choose green leafy vegetables or salad. You should eat fruit by itself on an empty stomach. Ideally, you should not eat any other food, particularly protein foods, for an hour before and after eating fruit.

On those days when you want to cheat and eat roasted meat and vegetables, or fish and chips, you can "food stack." This means eating the protein part of the meal first so that the concentrated hydrochloric acid juices in the stomach can break down the protein properly. Eat the starchier foods after this. Since starch digestion begins in the mouth, chew each mouthful thoroughly.

Food-combining Menu

This one-day meal plan provides an interesting and varied menu that follows the principles of food-combining.

- ◆ **Breakfast**
  half a papaya with the juice of $1/4$ lemon squeezed over and blueberries
- ◆ **Lunch** (carbohydrate meal)
  baked sweet potato with mixed vegetable salad
- ◆ **Dinner** (protein meal)
  baked salmon with green, leafy vegetables

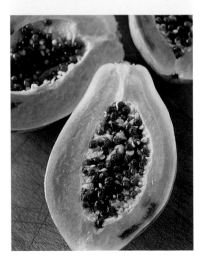

An Eastern Perspective

In Traditional Chinese Medicine (TCM) allergies are considered to be a reflection of poor digestion and a weakness of the Earth element. This element is associated with digestion and absorption, with the stomach and spleen/pancreas, and with the color yellow. A good practice, according to TCM, is to eat a nourishing breakfast when the stomach is in power (between 7 and 9 AM) and digestion is at its peak.

"WARMING" FOODS

In TCM, warming foods and herbs are considered highly beneficial in building the strength of the stomach and spleen/pancreas. You should include warming spices in your cooking, such as ginger, coriander seeds, and cardamom.

Some raw food in the diet is important for a rich supply of nutrients, but in the long term, if these foods are eaten all the time to the exclusion of others, they are thought to weaken "digestive fire" (a TCM term used to describe digestion). For this reason, you will not find copious amounts of salad recommended in level I because it can stimulate cleansing at too fast a pace (*see Anatomy of a Cleanse, pages 14–17*).

SUGAR CRAVINGS

Hypoglycemia, or low blood glucose levels, is a condition experienced mainly by people with diabetes. In TCM, hypoglycemia is a symptom of a weak spleen, causing a lack of energy coupled with a week spleen. Both the spleen and the sweet taste are connected, in TCM, with the Earth element. When the spleen is weak, an obsession with sweet food is common. Ensure that you have a good supply of complex carbohydrates such as brown rice and high-quality protein and keep your blood glucose levels stable by eating either three complete meals a day or six smaller ones.

Rather than trying to deny a craving for something sweet-tasting altogether, satisfy it by choosing sweetness from a natural source, such as:

- dates
- fruits rich in enzymes (papaya, kiwifruit, or pineapple)
- vegetables with a sweet taste, e.g., baked parsnips or sweet potatoes.

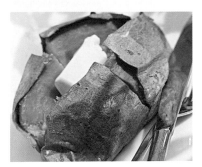

PROGRAM FOR LEVEL II

The theme of this level of the detox program is helping the body to "let go." The main focus is detoxing the colon, which benefits the digestive tract and also helps the skin and lungs discharge their toxins.

AIMS OF THE PROGRAM

The colon is the main section of the large intestine (bowel) and its lining is one of the body's most important defensive barriers against toxins. A poor diet of processed, low-fiber foods can damage the colon, in time leading to problems such as leaky gut syndrome (*see Glossary*). If damage is not

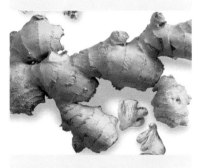

corrected, the whole immune system may eventually become undermined.

In level I, you improved your diet so that the colon is no longer being bombarded with unsuitable foods. The aim of this level is to repair the colon's lining and make the organ fully active

again. Cleansing the colon will benefit the appearance of the skin and improve your complexion.

Your Program

♦ Follow the dietary guidelines (*see pages 47–48*). These foods limit the damaging effects of free radicals and harmful bacteria, thus helping to repair the colon lining. Drink plenty of water.

♦ Continue to support digestion, a level I aim, with digestive enzymes (*see page 74*) and ginger (*see page 71*).

♦ Remove toxic waste material and bacteria, including parasites and *Candida*, from the colon (*see page 49–50*).

♦ Reduce exposure to new toxins (*see pages 51–52*).

♦ Repopulate the colon with probiotics (beneficial bowel flora) (*see page 52*).

♦ Every day, do the Breath of Life (*see page 100*) and the level II meditations (*see pages 110–111*).

♦ Practice the spa techniques for level II (*see pages 82–83*).

♦ For advice on how long to stay at level II, see page 20.

Food and Dietary Guidelines

Add these foods to the dietary program you began at level I (*see pages 40–1*).

- **Fiber-rich foods** Increase your consumption of these. The most important colon-cleansing material is vegetable and whole-grain fiber, which stimulates and enhances peristaltic action (the wavelike contractions of the colon that encourage proper elimination). In addition to vegetables, eat plenty of grains, including brown rice, millet, and quinoa (not, botanically, a true grain, but it can be used as one). These have lots of fiber and are gentle on the colon. Ideally, serve grains with the day's two main meals. Millet and quinoa taste rather bland and are best added to soups, or tossed into a stir-fry that includes plenty of garden herbs and spices.

- **Vegetables** Eat plenty at level II. They contain a high proportion of water and are also predominantly alkaline. To function healthily, the body's chemical balance needs to be slightly more alkaline than acid

and vegetables help counteract the effects of the many high-acid foods, such as meat and dairy products. Most vegetables are also rich in soluble fiber, which can reduce the absorption of toxic substances.

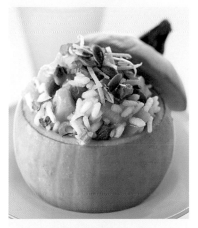

All vegetables contain protective phytochemicals, but cruciferous vegetables (brussels sprouts, cabbage, cauliflower, and broccoli), are particularly important. Include a varied mix of vegetables at each meal. (Arthritis sufferers should avoid the nightshade group of vegetables – potatoes, tomatoes, eggplant, and peppers).

- **Flax seeds** Sprinkle these nutritious seeds on cereals. They are a "complete protein," i.e. they contain all the essential amino acids, and they also have omega-3 fatty acids and small amounts of omega-6 acids, vitamins, and trace minerals. Flax seeds are a very useful source of fiber: they form a mucilaginous mass that helps to line the digestive tract and can heal inflammation.

On Waking

The body works well if its chemical balance is slightly alkaline. To alkanize the system, drink the juice of a lemon in warm water on rising. This helps activate the kidneys.

◆ **Protein** Reduce your protein intake at level II to ensure swift transit of food through the bowel (protein can slow this). Have protein three times a week, focusing on vegetable sources such as sprouted seeds. Sesame, pumpkin, and sunflower seeds are excellent sources of vegetable protein. Pumpkin seeds and oily fish are also thought to expel worms from the intestine.

◆ **Legumes** Eat plenty of fiber-rich legumes (lentils, beans, and soybean products). Before cooking, soak legumes overnight in filtered water with some lemon juice and kombu seaweed; this greatly increases their enzyme content and deactivates a substance that can cause indigestion and gas.

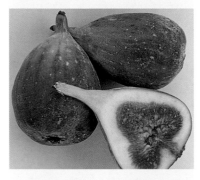

◆ **Gentle laxatives** Include foods such as prunes, figs, rhubarb, kale, parsley, and other green vegetables in the diet to ward off constipation.

◆ **Seaweed** Use this regularly in cooking for its detoxifying properties. It contains sodium alginate, which can bind toxic

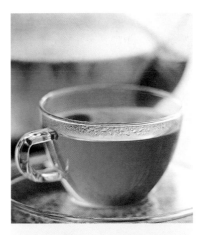

heavy metals and radioactive materials into harmless salts for elimination through the intestines. The seaweed wakame can aid the elimination of intestinal parasites.

◆ **Onions, garlic, and horseradish** The pungent flavor is connected to the Metal element so add these white pungent foods to your diet. They are natural antibiotics.

◆ **Cinnamon** Use this spice in cooking and add it to hot drinks. It is antibacterial and antiparasitic.

◆ **Green tea** This has phytochemicals, which demonstrate antibacterial, antiviral, and anticancer properties. It is also preferable because it has less caffeine than black tea.

◆ **Ginger** Add grated fresh ginger to hot water for digestive support.

◆ **Caution** Avoid fruit at level II as its naturally high sugar content may exacerbate fungal infections. (*See also Candida, page 50.*)

Supplements for Level II

◆ **Aloe vera juice** This provides several benefits at level II. It stimulates movement of waste through the colon and repairs the damaged, leaky colon wall, so that fewer toxins are able to enter. Take 0.34–1.01 fl.oz a day of whole leaf aloe vera juice (use the 99.7 percent pure version).

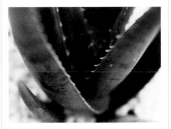

◆ **Psyllium seed husks** This is a useful cleansing supplement at level II. The husks add bulk and speed the transit of food through the intestines. They help lift impacted material and some harmful bacteria off the colon wall. Psyllium husks must be taken with plenty of water to allow the fibers to swell up. You should follow the manufacturer's instructions, taking 2–4 1,000-mg capsules a day with 20 fl. oz. (600 ml) water 2 hours after food. The ideal intake of psyllium depends on your body size, so start low and increase the dosage until the desired affect is achieved.

◆ **Combination supplements** You can find formulas that contain psyllium together with other cleansing herbs and bentonite clay, which helps absorb old toxins from the colon.

Colonic Irrigation

After two or three weeks at level II, when hardened material in the colon has been loosened, it may be useful to go to a trained professional for a few sessions of colonic irrigation to remove impacted feces. This will ensure that toxins in it are not reabsorbed.

Naturopaths often prescribe water, herbal, and even organic coffee enemas (to stimulate the liver to detox); discuss all these with a qualified practitioner before you undertake them.

Colonic irrigation is not for everyone. For example, Traditional Chinese Medicine does not advise it for someone who is very weak. Before trying colonic irrigation, consult your doctor about its value for you.

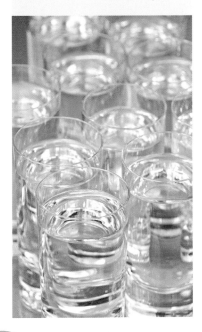

Dealing with Parasites

Parasites, especially worms, are a common cause of damage to the colon lining, reducing nutrient absorption and weakening the immune system. Symptoms include bloating, abdominal pain, irregular bowel habits, chronic fatigue, and food sensitivities. Olive leaf, golden seal, and garlic are useful herbs. However, if you suspect parasites, it is advisable that you seek professional advice since there are more potent herbs

Candida Infections

Candida albicans is a fungus naturally present in the body that can flourish too strongly when there is digestive imbalance. Taking the contraceptive pill or several courses of antibiotics can

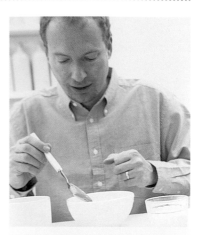

also cause it to multiply out of control. It results in infections such as vaginal and oral thrush and candidiasis. The measures in level I of the program begin to correct the problem and the more stringent measures in level II can help to clear it up.
Caution Do not eat fruit if you have a candida problem; the fungus thrives on sugar. Also avoid mushrooms, products with yeast (e.g., bread, pizza), alcohol, smoked foods, and fermented products such as soy sauce.

Candida Symptoms

- Constant fatigue; cravings for carbohydrates and sweet foods caused by lowered blood glucose levels.

- Fungal infections, such as thrush, cystitis, and anal itching, or skin infections such as ringworm or athlete's foot.

- Weakened digestive function with bloating after eating, irritable bowel syndrome.

- Generally not feeling well, poor concentration, aches and pains, and heightened sensitivity to environmental toxins such as exhaust fumes or tobacco.

Probiotics

At the end of an intestinal cleansing program the bowel must be returned to proper functioning and the intestinal tract repopulated with beneficial or "friendly" bacteria. Probiotics, which are natural bacteria used to encourage the development of friendly organisms, do this. The beneficial bacteria *Lactobacillus acidophilus* and *Bifidobacteria* are probiotics that are able to metabolize vitamins and hormones, neutralize drugs and carcinogens, and inhibit the growth of parasites, viruses, fungi, and toxic bacteria.

People with chronic intestinal disorders such as irritable bowel syndrome (IBS) are advised to use supplements that provide between 5–10 billion beneficial bacteria per capsule. These are taken two to three times a day for a minimum of two weeks to shift unwanted organisms and repopulate the intestinal tract with beneficial types. *Acidophilus* produces the enzyme lactase, so increasing digestion of lactose (milk sugar). It should be one with scientifically proven therapeutic qualities that allows beneficial bacteria to adhere to the intestinal wall and inhibits the growth of harmful bacteria. It should also be made in a way that ensures its potency survives in the gastrointestinal tract.

Reducing Exposure to Environmental Toxins

An important part of level II detox is to reduce exposure to toxins. Many environmental toxins can be tackled and exposure to them considerably reduced.

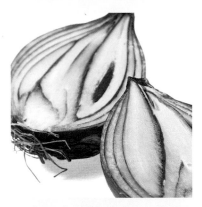

Providing probiotics

◆ Eat live yogurt, which contains varying amounts of probiotic organisms that can heal the intestines and reduce bowel toxicity.

◆ Eat fibers called fructo-oligosaccharides (FOS). Found in onions and asparagus, these are "prebiotics" that feed the beneficial probiotic bacteria. They are also essential at this repopulation stage because they help stop parasitic bacteria and toxins from attaching themselves to the walls of the intestine.

◆ Take a probiotic supplement in the third and fourth weeks of the level II program.

◆ Choose household cleaning products that are natural and environment-friendly. Recent

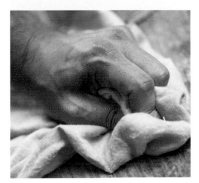

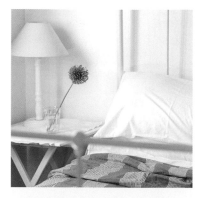

research has found that many laundry and cleaning products contain pollutants, irritants, and carcinogens that can cause a range of symptoms including nausea and skin disorders.

◆ Minimize exposure to chemicals at home and at work. Check there are no leaks from gas appliances and keep dust and mold to a minimum. Mold can aggravate fungal infections.

◆ When cleaning, use hot water and natural products such as baking soda and borax. Olive oil makes a good furniture polish.

◆ When you buy clothes, look for natural fabrics such as cotton, wool, linen, and silk.

◆ Do not use antiperspirants and deodorants containing toxic metals, such as aluminum, and choose body lotions and cosmetics that are as natural as possible, bearing in mind that these are absorbed through the skin. Without chemical-laden products

your skin will begin to smell "sweeter" as your body becomes cleaner, but in the meantime, wash more frequently with soap and water.

◆ Where possible, and with your doctor's advice, find a natural alternative to any over-the-counter drugs or medications you have been prescribed. Nonsteroidal anti-inflammatory drugs (NSAIDs) are the most common nonbacterial cause of damage to the colon.

◆ Pesticides and chemicals used in modern farming practices can be very harmful to the colon,

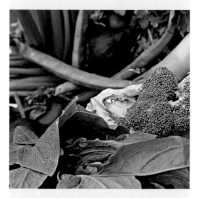

immune system, and liver. Buy organic vegetables and other produce where possible and wash nonorganic produce in both cider vinegar and water.

◆ In the kitchen, use stainless steel, glass, or earthenware. Avoid non-stick pans, or those made with aluminum and copper, which can leach metals into foods.

An Eastern Perspective

In Traditional Chinese Medicine (TCM), the lungs, large intestine, and skin are the partner organs for the Metal element (*see page 33*). The lungs expel carbon dioxide and the large intestine eliminates solid residues, while the skin is regarded as "the third lung" for expelling waste.

If waste is not eliminated from the body efficiently, it can have an adverse effect on the skin as well as on the digestive system. Toxins that remain in the colon for too long will be discharged through the skin. The Chinese believe the best time to have a bowel movement is 5–7 am (the time of the large intestine according to the TCM body clock). Following such a regime may help regulate the bowel.

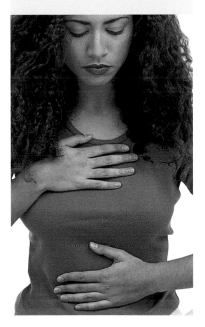

The color white is associated with the Metal element in TCM and, according to practitioners, a pale skin is indicative of lung problems. The breathing exercises (*see page 100*) that are part of this program will help the lungs to function at optimum levels. Breathing is one of the primary ways in which the body and its energy levels are replenished. Because breathing is so simple and so basic to life, its significance to well-being is often overlooked until specific symptoms – shortness of breath or wheezing, for example – begin to impede breathing.

Practitioners of TCM believe that the highest function of the lungs is to be the "Receiver of Energy" bringing *qi* (vital energy) from inhaled air into the body where it is combined with food *qi* from the spleen (an Earth element organ worked on in level I).

The lungs govern the breath and are responsible for the production of defensive *qi* (referred to as *wei qi*), which is believed to protect the body from invading negative environmental changes and harmful bacteria. If the lungs are weak, the body will be more prone to infections because resistance is lowered. Therefore, it is important to strengthen the lungs during level II of the detox program.

PROGRAM FOR LEVEL III

In the previous two levels, the body was nourished and the superficial detox organs were cleansed. This final level of the body detox program concentrates on the liver and kidneys – the deep organs of detoxification.

AIMS OF THE PROGRAM

The liver and kidneys detoxify harmful compounds in a two-step procedure, which can easily go out of balance. The aim of level III is to restore the proper functioning of the liver and kidneys by eating particularly helpful foods and supplements and by reducing exposure to harmful toxins.

How the Liver Works

The liver detoxifies substances in two distinct phases. The kidneys eliminate toxins after the liver has metabolized them.

Phase I In this phase, the liver uses a group of enzymes called cytochrome P450s to neutralize some toxins immediately and convert others into water-soluble forms that the kidneys can then eliminate. Some toxins, however, are only partially processed at this stage and are converted to forms called "reactive intermediates."

Your Program

- ◆ Ensure that the diet includes the right nutrients and herbs (*see pages 56–57*).
- ◆ Take antioxidants to help the liver's enzymes (*see page 57*).
- ◆ Take supplements to help production of glutathione (*see page 57*).
- ◆ Reduce exposure to toxins (*see opposite*).
- ◆ Do breathing exercises and the meditations for level III (*see pages 112–13*)
- ◆ Follow the spa techniques for level III (*see pages 84–85*).
- ◆ See page 21 for how long to spend at level III.

Phase II In phase II, enzymes in the liver attach chemicals to the reactive intermediates to neutralize them or to make them easy to excrete in the urine or bile. If phase II is not working properly and the reactive intermediates are not flushed out, they remain in the body where they can cause damage.

Any imbalance between phase I and phase II can lead to an

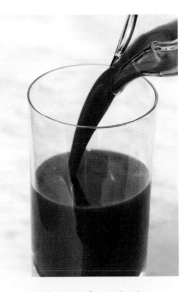

accumulation of reactive inter-mediates. The buildup increases free-radical damage and causes symptoms such as nausea, fatigue, headaches, confusion, depression, and anxiety.

Healing Crisis

Toxins are often stored in fatty tissue. When this begins to break down during level III, the toxins are released, causing discomfort – the healing crisis. It is not unusual to feel that you must eat comfort food at this stage. This is because the body's protective mechanism kicks in and tries to redeposit or "encapsulate" toxins in fat cells. This may alleviate symptoms in the short term, but it also increases fatty deposits and toxic load. Rather than reaching for chocolate, you should eat foods

that aid phase II liver enzymes in their job of removing reactive intermediates. Such foods include proteins, which bind to toxins, and fruit, vegetables, and juices that contain substances that are vital for the liver's production of glutathione, an important antioxidant. The foods that provide the right essential nutrients are included in the dietary guidelines on pages 56–57. You should also reduce your exposure to dietary and environmental toxins (*see below*).

Essential Dietary and Environmental Changes

◆ Remove alcohol, tobacco, caffeine, saturated fats, barbecued/charred meats, and burned toast from the diet.

◆ Avoid foods that are highly reactive, such as cow's milk and wheat, or foods containing yeast until such time as the main benefits of detoxification have occurred. Replace them with suitable alternatives (*see page 39*).

◆ Reduce exposure to vehicle exhaust and paint fumes.

◆ Avoid inhaling dioxins, found in solvents such as dry-cleaning fluids or bleaches.

◆ Reduce exposure to organophosphate fertilizers, pesticides, and herbicides.

◆ Ideally, reduce intake of medicines, including steroid hormones and anti-inflammatory drugs (NSAIDs), but only under the strict supervision of your doctor.

Food and Dietary Guidelines

Eating the right foods can help phase II liver enzymes eliminate reactive intermediates from the body. You should add the following foods to those you were eating in level II of the program.

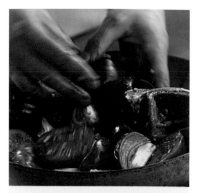

- **Phytonutrient-rich foods** The following are rich in substances that aid detoxification and protect the body: cruciferous vegetables, such as broccoli (flavonoids, indole-3 carbinol, vitamin C), lemons (limonene), red grapes (ellagic acid in skin and seeds), garlic (diallyl sulfides), soy (isoflavones), rosemary (carnosol), and turmeric (curcumin).

- **Sour-tasting foods** Foods that taste sour stimulate liver function. Lemon juice in hot water is a good cleansing drink. Citrus fruits are aggressive cleansers and should be avoided in the previous two levels. However, at level III try grapefruit juice: the flavanone naringenin in grapefruit helps alleviate a healing crisis because

it slows down production of reactive intermediates.

- **Antioxidant superfoods** Eat plenty of the following to protect the liver: tomatoes (lycopene), watercress (isothiocyanate), carrots (beta-carotene), peppers (beta-cryptoxanthin), beets (beta-carotene, vitamin C), and berries (anthocyanins).

- **Protein** Have some protein daily. Choose from lean meat, eggs, or soy. Protein is essential for proper phase II detoxification because it provides key amino acids that bind to toxins and neutralize their toxicity.

- **Foods rich in B vitamins** These help the functioning of phase II enzymes: green vegetables (folic acid), lean meat (vitamin B_{12}), wheat germ (vitamin B_6), and eggs (choline).

- **Foods containing sulfur** Sulfur in garlic, onions, red peppers, brussels sprouts, egg yolk, and broccoli aid phase II enzymes.

Gentle Detox Mixture

For a gentle, effective daily detox mixture, mix the juice of 1 lemon with 2 tablespoons of flax seed oil. Add 1 teaspoon grated ginger, a pinch of cayenne, and 1 crushed garlic clove. If you cannot stomach this mixture as a drink, use it as a dressing for a green salad.

◆ **Fresh juices** Make these with lemon, carrot, ginger, and apple. The pectin in apples promotes bile secretion and interrupts the production of cholesterol in the liver. A juice of beets and celery or watercress juice diluted 50:50 with filtered water, taken morning and afternoon, stimulates cleansing. Add wheat grass to juices for extra nutrients.

◆ **Bitter greens** Dandelion, chicory, radicchio, and watercress, combined with a dressing based on the gentle detox mixture (*see box, page 56*), help stimulate the liver and gallbladder.

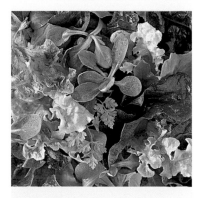

Supplements to Support Detoxification

The following supplements should be incorporated into the diet to support the activity of the phase I and II liver enzymes.

◆ Glutathione is an antioxidant crucial for the liver. It helps the organ excrete toxins such as exhaust fumes, tobacco smoke, radiation, chemicals, and drugs.

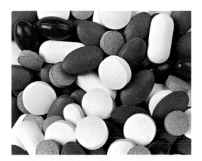

Take 250–500 mg twice daily. Also, look for supplements containing cysteine, methionine, taurine, lysine, and glutamine. These all boost the body's own production of glutathione.

◆ Antioxidant supplements are essential for phase II detoxification (*see box below*)

◆ B vitamins, including vitamin B_{12}, folic acid, and B_1, B_2, B_3, and B_6 are also necessary. The best way to take them is in the form of a B-complex or multivitamin to support liver detoxification and boost underactive pathways.

Antioxidants for Level III

Unless otherwise stated, take all of these antioxidant supplements once a day.

◆ **Vitamin A** 12,500 iu
◆ **Vitamin C** 500 mg twice daily
◆ **Vitamin E** 600 iu
◆ **Selenium** 150 mcg
◆ **Zinc** 25 mg
◆ **Copper** 5 mg
◆ **Manganese** 10 mg
◆ **Coenzyme Q10** 10 mg
◆ **Milk thistle** 120–160 mg three times a day.

An Eastern Perspective

The liver and gallbladder are closely related: the liver produces bile, which is stored in the gallbladder until it is needed to break down fats. In Traditional Chinese Medicine (TCM), the liver and gallbladder are also closely connected. They are partner organs and are associated with the Wood element (*see the Five Elements Table, page 33*).

LIVER AND BLOOD

One of the key functions of the liver according to TCM is filtering and storing blood. The Chinese believe that it is important to be in bed before this function begins (they say it takes place at 11 pm and 3 am) because, for it to happen effectively, the body needs to be horizontal and resting so that the blood is not diverted to other sites. In TCM, if the liver is unable to store, release, and purify the blood, stagnation of qi (vital energy) can follow. This stagnation manifests as increased levels of both physical and mental tension and a tendency to wake unrefreshed and tired in the morning.

COLORS, SEASONS, AND TASTES

Green is the color of the Wood element and, in TCM, a green tinge on the face is considered a indication of liver imbalance. It is the color people turn if feeling nauseous (another symptom indicating a Wood element imbalance). Green is also seen abundantly in springtime, the season associated with the liver and gallbladder .

The taste connected to the Wood element is sour, thus lemon with its sour taste supports these organs. Lemon has the added benefit of being a rich source of limonene, a key phytochemical necessary for the liver's phase II detoxification.

THE KIDNEYS

The kidneys play a key role in detoxification, since large portions of the body's wastes are eliminated through them. They also help remove poisons from the liver. In both Western medicine and TCM, the kidneys and bladder are connected both structurally and functionally. Considered by practitioners of TCM to be the "water gateway" of the body, the bladder acts as a container for the urine released by the kidneys.

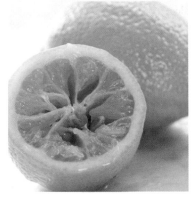

LEVEL I: PROTEIN

Strengthens and supports the spleen ◆ Helps reduce cravings ◆ Builds *qi* energy

EGGS

In addition to being an excellent protein source, eggs are rich in vitamins (especially A, B complex, D, and E) and minerals (including zinc and iron in the yolk), and the

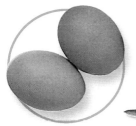

amino acids methionine and cysteine. Egg yolks contain lecithin, the choline that plays an important role in many metabolic functions, including fat metabolism, making it ideal for the level I detox. Egg yolks contain cholesterol, but recent research shows that this does not increase blood cholesterol. World Health Organization guidelines state up to ten eggs may be safely eaten each week (including eggs in baking and desserts).

> DETOX BENEFITS
> ◆ Excellent source of high-quality protein
> ◆ Contain amino acids that support detoxification

OILY FISH

The oil in deep-water oily fish such as tuna, salmon, mackerel, herrings, and sardines contains omega-3 essential fatty acids, which are vital for healthy cell function, for moving fats around the body, and for reducing inflammation. During detox, they can

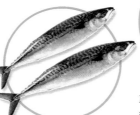

help reduce cravings and food allergies. Omega-3 fatty acids are not made in the body so they must be supplied in the food we eat, and yet they are one of the main nutrients missing in modern diets. A diet high in omega-3 essential fatty acids helps reduce heart disease and protects against some forms of cancer. Aim to eat 3–5 portions of oily fish a week during level I of the detox program.

> DETOX BENEFITS
> ◆ Helps reduce cravings and food allergies
> ◆ Rich in omega-3 essential fatty acids

LAMB

Lamb is one of the most pure and least allergenic of all meats, which is why it is the mainstay of the well-known lamb and pear allergy diet. Traditional Chinese

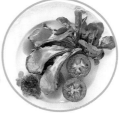

Medicine sees red meat as a good tonic for the blood and a strengthener of *qi* (energy). Lamb is a very good source of protein, most of the B vitamins, zinc, and an easily assimilated form of iron. It is high in saturated fats and calories, so choose lean cuts such as fillet or leg, or remove as much fat as possible before cooking. Include up to three servings of lamb in your diet every week in this stage of your detox.

> DETOX BENEFITS
> ◆ Nonallergenic
> ◆ Good blood tonic
> ◆ Good source of zinc and iron
> ◆ Build's *qi* (energy)

LEVEL I: SPROUTS

Nourish the body with easy-to-absorb nutrients

◆ Support the digestive system ◆ Antioxidant effect

Sprouting seeds and beans "predigest" their nutrients, making them easier for the body to absorb. They are superfoods with a high protein, enzyme, vitamin, and mineral content. Sprouted beans produce much less intestinal gas than whole beans and when potentially allergenic grains such as wheat are sprouted they do not cause an allergenic reaction. All these qualities make sprouted beans and seeds ideal for level I detox with its emphasis on nourishing the body.

MUNG BEANS
These are probably the most commonly sprouted beans (they are

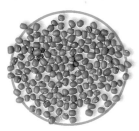

a favorite ingredient in Chinese dishes). Sprouted mung beans contain powerful phytochemicals including coumestrol, which studies have shown to be antioxidant as well as anti-inflammatory.

These sprouts may also protect against cancer and moderate the negative effects of the hormone estrogen.

DETOX BENEFITS
◆ Easy for body to absorb
◆ Nourishing sources of protein, enzymes, vitamins, and minerals

ALFALFA SEEDS
Sharing the positive benefits of mung beans, sprouted alfalfa seeds

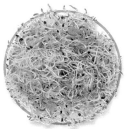

also have beneficial effects on the digestive system. They contain isoflavones that have similar properties to the female hormone estrogen.

DETOX BENEFITS
◆ Easy for body to absorb
◆ Support the digestive system

PUMPKIN SEEDS
The sprouted seeds of the pumpkin are particularly rich in zinc, a mineral essential for normal growth, development, immunity, and fertility.

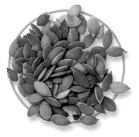

Pumpkin seeds are also a good source of protein, fiber, magnesium, phosphorus, potassium, and iron. They contain phytosterols, which can lower cholesterol and inhibit cancer development.

DETOX BENEFITS
◆ Nourish the body at level I with a wide range of nutrients
◆ Good source of vitamins, fiber, and omega-3 fats
◆ Provide rich supply of several minerals, especially zinc, and key plant nutrients

● CAUTION
Avoid all bean sprouts if you have lupus because they may cause a reaction.

LEVEL I: VEGETABLES

Powerful source of antioxidants that neutralize toxins

Strengthen digestive function ◆ Boost *qi* (energy)

SWEET POTATO

The orange fleshed sweet potato gets its color from the carotenoid beta-carotene, a powerful antioxidant that is converted to vitamin A in the liver. Beta-carotene is able to render harmless free radicals, which are the toxic byproducts of metabolism and pollution. If left unattended, free radicals may damage cells and start cancerous changes. Both the creamy and orange-fleshed varieties of sweet

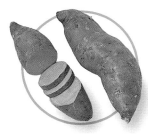

potatoes are rich in carbohydrates, potassium, and vitamins C and E. Traditional Chinese Medicine believes sweet potatoes warm the stomach, strengthen the internal organs, and support *qi* (energy).

DETOX BENEFITS
◆ Rich in toxin-neutralizing beta-carotene
◆ Source of antioxidants

FENNEL

Practitioners of Traditional Chinese Medicine consider fennel to be an energy booster that tonifies yang energy and thus strengthens the body. The volatile oils and flavonoids in fennel support the proper functioning of the digestive system and reduce gas. Fennel also

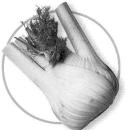

improves the function of the spleen. Fennel seeds have a strong diuretic action and drinking fennel tea helps reduce sugar cravings. This, coupled with its ability to help the body eliminate fats and its low calorie content, makes fennel a helpful aid in a weight-loss program.

DETOX BENEFITS
◆ Supports digestive system
◆ Boosts *qi* (energy)

● **CAUTION**
Do not eat fennel seeds during pregnancy.

TOMATO

In Traditional Chinese Medicine (TCM), tomatoes are used as a tonic to the digestive system and to help alkalize the blood, making them a valuable addition to your level I detox diet. They are a rich source of lycopene, a fat-soluble carotenoid responsible for their red color. Research suggests that the most important antioxidant, lycopene, plays an important part in the prevention of a variety

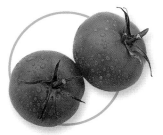

of diseases, including certain cancers. Eating tomatoes with oil such as olive or flax increases the body's ability to absorb lycopene by 70 percent.

DETOX BENEFITS
◆ Source of the most potent antioxidant, lycopene
◆ TCM digestive tonic

● **CAUTION**
Tomatoes are known to aggravate canker sores and rheumatoid arthritis.

LEVEL I: FRUIT

Packed with nutrients and fiber ◆ Full of toxin-neutralizing
antioxidants ◆ Help control blood glucose levels

Nutritionists have long recommended eating five portions of different fruit and vegetables every day. Level I of the detox program aims to support and nourish the body. Certain fruits, with their wide range of nutrients and other constitutents, are particularly suitable.

PINEAPPLE

Bromelain, an enzyme in pineapple, has strong anti-inflammatory and protein-digesting properties. Although the fresh fruit contains only small amounts of the enzyme, some studies suggest it can still help digestion and assimilation of nutrients, making it a good choice of fruit to

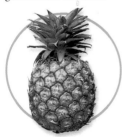

include in your level I detox. In Traditional Chinese Medicine (TCM) the pineapple's yellow color is associated with the Earth element, which is connected to the digestive system.

DETOX BENEFITS
◆ Digestive aid that may help body assimilate nutrients
◆ Believed in TCM to help digestion

BERRIES

Both the firm types of berries, such as black-berries and blackcurrants, and the soft types, such as raspberries, are rich in

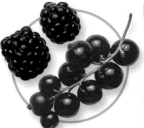

antioxidants, flavonoids, and anthocyanins, which help neutralize toxic-free radicals (*see Glossary*). Bilberries and blueberries, which are very rich in antioxidants, are also said to stabilize blood glucose levels and alleviate hypoglycemia (low blood glucose), a key objective of level I detox.

DETOX BENEFITS
◆ Rich in antioxidants that help to neutralize toxins
◆ Can help stabilize blood glucose levels

PEAR

Pears are known to be one of the few foods that are unlikely to cause an intolerance or an allergic reaction. Since they also help to control blood-sugar levels, they are invaluable in level I detox. Pears are also a good

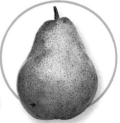

source of antioxidants and pectin, a form of soluble fiber that can remove heavy metal from the body and lower cholesterol levels. To get maximum nutritional value from pears, eat them whole (after washing): eating the skin ensures that you benefit from the valuable fiber and the antioxidant hydroxycinnamic acids, which are thought to block the formation of cancer-causing agents.

DETOX BENEFITS
◆ Hypoallergenic
◆ Fiber, antioxidants
◆ Regulates blood glucose

LEVEL II: GRAINS

Speed up transit of food through the colon ◆ Easily digested ◆ Help expel toxins ◆ Low risk of allergy

RICE

A gluten-free grain, rice is considered to be one of the least allergenic foods available. Try to include it in your diet frequently

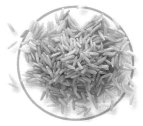

during level II for its many health-giving properties. In addition to being a vital source of protein, rice provides a gentle form of fiber that increases the peristaltic action (wavelike contractions) of the colon, helping to hasten the transit of stools and thus reducing the time toxins stay in the colon. Because rice absorbs water during cooking, it contains plenty of moisture, which can help prevent dehydration in the intestine and so relieve constipation. The grain is rich in the amino acids methionine and cysteine. The latter can increase the ease with which mucus is eliminated from the lungs and helps protect lung tissue.

DETOX BENEFITS
◆ Hypoallergenic
◆ Good source of cleansing fiber
◆ Helps keep blood-glucose levels steady
◆ Prevents constipation

MILLET

One of the oldest cultivated cereals known, millet is an alkaline, gluten-free grain. It contains seven of the eight essential amino acids and is thus a very good source of protein. Because, like rice, it is

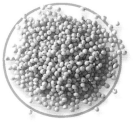

gluten-free, it is easily digested (gluten can irritate the walls of the intestine and many people find it hard to digest). Also in millet's favor in level II is that it is a gentle form of fiber.

DETOX BENEFITS
◆ Easily digested carbohydrate
◆ The best source of protein of the grains

QUINOA AND AMARANTH

Quinoa, the mother food of the Incas, is an easily digested, cleansing food that is a good source of protein and nutrients, including vitamins B and E, and minerals, such as calcium and iron.

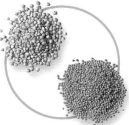

Amaranth is another very ancient grain that has a low allergy risk. It is a concentrated source of protein and other nutrients, such as calcium, magnesium, silicon, and the amino acid lysine.

DETOX BENEFITS
◆ Easily digested and cleansing
◆ Hypoallergenic
◆ Packed with nutrients

● NOTE
To increase their nutritional value, soak all grains for 24 hours before cooking. Drain, then bring to the boil in fresh water.

LEVEL II: VEGETABLES

Stimulate the immune system ◆ Protect against free-radical damage ◆ Antiviral and antibacterial properties

CARROT

An exceptionally rich source of the potent antioxidant beta-carotene, carrots contain most of

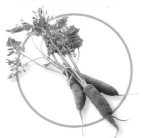

the vitamins and minerals, iron, and calcium needed by the body in an easily assimilated form. Carrots are said to eliminate putrefactive bacteria in the colon; they also contain an essential oil that helps fight the fungal infection, ringworm. Carrots stimulate the immune system and can facilitate the elimination of intestinal parasites. They are also antibacterial: able, for instance, to fight the listeria bacteria that cause food poisoning.

DETOX BENEFITS
◆ Antibacterial effect on the bacteria in food
◆ Rich source of toxin-neutralizing beta-carotene

KALE (COLLARD GREENS)

A member of the cabbage family, kale contains phytonutrients that help support detoxification and has the highest overall antioxidant ability of leafy green vegetables, the highest concentration of beta-carotene being found in the darker green leaves. It is rich in indole-3 carbinol that specifically protects against hormone-mediated

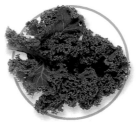

cancers, and studies have linked regular intake of leafy green vegetables to a reduced risk of cancers, including colon cancer. It is also a rich source of calcium.

DETOX BENEFITS
◆ Highest antioxidant ability of all leafy green vegetables
◆ Phytonutrients support detoxification

ONION

Onions are rich in the antioxidant quercetin that protects against free radical damage. Onions are valuable in your level II detox for the

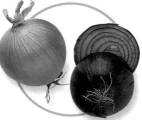

fructo-oligosaccharides (FOS) they contain. These enhance the activity of beneficial bacteria in the gut, so helping to fight fungal infections such as those caused by *Candida* overgrowth. Onions also contain flavonoids that have been shown to have an antiviral action and can also inhibit the replication of viruses. To retain their high quercetin levels, eat onions raw or lightly cooked in olive oil.

DETOX BENEFITS
◆ Rich in the antioxidant quercetin
◆ Antimicrobial and enhance healthy gut microflora

LEVEL II: SUPERFOODS

Cleanse the lymphatic system ◆ Expel waste from the body

Purify the blood ◆ Cleanse the gastrointestinal tract

SEAWEEDS

Do not underestimate the value of seaweeds during your level II detox. Their soothing, healing proper-

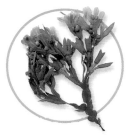

ties fortify the immune system and the gastro-intestinal tract. They are good sources of protein and soluble fiber and have a very high mineral content. High levels of iodine and selenium make them strongly antioxidant too. Traditional Chinese Medicine (TCM) uses seaweed to improve the body's water metabolism, clean up the lymphatic system, and alkalinize the blood. Nori, wakame, and kombu are the best varieties to try initially.

DETOX BENEFITS
◆ Fortify the gastrointestinal tract
◆ Strongly antioxidant
◆ Cleanse lymphatic system in TCM

WATERCRESS

The peppery taste of watercress is caused by a benzyl mustard oil (also present in nasturtium leaves), a powerful antibiotic that is beneficial to the colon and intestinal flora. Watercress purifies the blood and expels metabolic acids and wastes from the body, so eating plenty of it enhances natural resistance and helps detoxify the body. It is exceptionally rich in

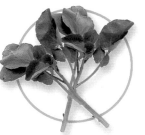

minerals, including calcium and iron, beta-carotene, and vitamin C. It also contains the phytochemical isothiocyanate, which can detoxify cancer-causing substances.

DETOX BENEFITS
◆ Expels waste from the body
◆ Benefits color and intestinal flora

SALAD GREENS

Containing vitamin C, beta-carotene, flavonols, and folic acid as well as fiber, salad leaves have rich cancer-protective effects. Mix salad greens

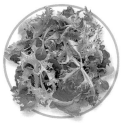

to benefit from the different phytochemicals: Romaine lettuce contains zeaxanthin, an important antioxidant phytochemical; lollo rosso is ten times richer in quercetin than other lettuce, giving it supreme antioxidant properties. Chicory detoxifies and cleanses the digestive tract and is high in fructo-oligosaccharides (FOS) that enhance the activity of beneficial bacteria in the gut.

DETOX BENEFITS
◆ Supreme antioxidants
◆ Cleanse digestive tract

LEVEL II: BOWELFOODS

Encourage beneficial bacteria in the intestines

Antiviral and antibacterial ◆ Reduce fungal infections

YOGURT

It has long been known that yogurt disables and kills bacteria, but now research shows that the probiotics (*Bifidobacterium*

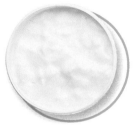

bifidum and *Lactobacillus acidophilus*) in live yogurt inhibit the formation of cancer-causing compounds, enhancing the immune system. The probiotics help the detox process by reducing inflammation and facilitating the elimination of intestinal parasites that cause damage to the gut wall. Yogurt should be eaten daily. Over a long time, yogurt increases gamma interferon, an immune-enhancing protein that stops viruses from reproducing. If you have intestinal irregularities, take a probiotic supplement.

DETOX BENEFITS
◆ Disables bacteria
◆ Enhances immune system

ASPARAGUS

The many active phyto-chemicals in asparagus (especially in the green variety), plus its pungent taste, which is associated with the Metal element in Traditional Chinese Medicine (TCM), make it a superb detox food. The main nutrients, including asparagines and potassium, help the detox process because they are diuretic, that is they eliminate excess water. Asparagus contains fructo-oligosaccharides (FOS), a form of fiber

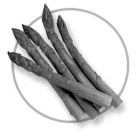

that promotes the growth of beneficial bacteria in the colon and inhibits the growth of colon cancer cells. In TCM asparagus is used to clear lung congestion and flush out the kidneys.

DETOX BENEFITS
◆ Diuretic effect
◆ Helps maintain healing bacteria in the intestines

FLAX SEEDS

High in soluble fiber, flax seeds assist in the removal of excess *Candida* bacteria from the intestine. They also slow down the release of sugars into the intestine, so the *Candida* bacteria have less to feed on

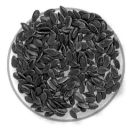

and cannot increase as rapidly. Flax seeds assist in the elimination of excess estrogen from the body and reduce the risk of certain cancers by lowering the amounts of circulating estrogens that stimulate the breast, cervical, and uterus tissue to divide. In addition, lignans, a phytonutrient found in flax seeds, have antiviral, antifungal, antibacterial, and even anticancer properties.

DETOX BENEFITS
◆ Inhibit growth of *Candida*
◆ Help reduce risk of certain cancers

LEVEL III: FRUIT

Stimulate detox enzymes ◆ Cleanse the liver and kidneys

◆ Help the body excrete toxic metals

LEMON

The peel and the inner parts of the lemon have the highest concentrations of phytochemicals. These include limonene and

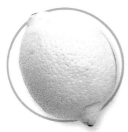

other limonoids that have the ability to stimulate both phase I and phase II enzymes, which are part of the liver's detoxification process (*see page 54*).

The vitamin C in lemons helps the body maintain the immune system. Lemons have a sour taste, a flavor that is associated with the Wood element and the liver in Traditional Chinese Medicine (TCM). They can benefit the liver in level III of the detox program: each morning, to help release liver stagnation, drink hot water with the grated zest and juice of half a lemon added. When juicing, use the whole fruit, to benefit from the flesh (the *yin* part) and the pith and skin (the *yang* parts).

> **DETOX BENFFITS**
> ◆ Stimulates detox enzymes
> ◆ Helps release liver stagnation

APPLE

Naturopaths value apples for their cleansing properties and ability to eliminate excess fluid and toxins from the body by acting on the kidneys. In level III, juice combinations containing apples have cleansing powers. Apples contain malic and tartaric acids, which aid the digestion of rich,

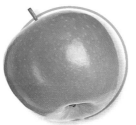

fatty foods that can weaken the liver. They are rich in pectin, a soluble fiber that can bind heavy metals such as lead and mercury and excrete them along with cholesterol.

> **DETOX BENEFITS**
> ◆ Cleansing for the kidneys and liver
> ◆ Helps excrete heavy metals and cholesterol

CRANBERRY

Apart from being a rich source of flavonoids, vitamins, and minerals, cranberries have the proven ability to remove harmful bacteria from the kidneys and bladder, and have been found to be far more potent at

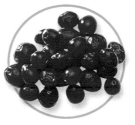

destroying urinary tract bacteria than conventional antibiotics. In fact, research has shown that a glass of cranberry juice is ten times as effective at killing urinary bacteria as conventional antibiotics. This is due to the cranberry's high percentage of mannose, a type of sugar that blocks the sites to which the bacteria adhere in the urinary tract, effectively flushing them out of the system.

> **DETOX BENFFITS**
> ◆ Remove harmful bacteria from bladder
> ◆ Rich source of antioxidants

LEVEL III: OILS

Strongly antioxidant ◆ Revive stress-weakened endocrine

and immune systems ◆ Support the kidneys

FLAX SEED OIL

The omega-3 essential fatty acids in flax seed oil regulate numerous metabolic functions and increase the body's ability

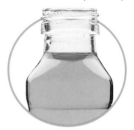

to metabolize oxygen. These fatty acids are also useful at this stage of your detox because they help the kidneys excrete excess water, and support the endocrine and immune systems that are so often weakened by stress. At this level, include oils such as flax seed in your diet every day: mix them into salad dressings or add to juices. For the best results, use a blend of unrefined organic flax seed, sunflower, and sesame oils. These provide omega-6 essential fatty acids that the body needs as well as omega-3 acids.

DETOX BENEFITS
- ◆ Helps kidneys excrete excess water
- ◆ Supports endocrine and immune systems

OLIVE OIL

The longevity and health associated with the diets of the Mediterranean region have long been attributed to olive oil. Research indicates it has a significant antioxidant action and prevents cholesterol from being oxidized into a harmful form that can cause heart disease. This mono-unsaturated oil is good for cooking since, unlike most polyunsaturated oils (safflower, sunflower, or soy), when heated, it is not easily oxidized to

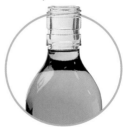

form damaging free radicals. Try to use extra-virgin olive oil, which, because it is less refined, contains larger quantities of the phytochemicals that are important in maintaining good health.

DETOX BENEFITS
- ◆ Significant antioxidant activity
- ◆ Stops cholesterol be-coming a free radical

SESAME OIL

Sesame oil contains a high percentage of healthy monounsaturated oils (oleic acid) along with omega-6 fatty acids. It is a key source of calcium and of phytic acid, which has antioxidant properties

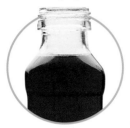

and boosts immunity. Sesame seeds and the oil from them contain a phytochemical called sesaminol. A powerful anti-inflammatory, it helps reduce pain. It also enhances the action of vitamin E and inhibits the absorption of dietary cholesterol. Use the oil in stir-fries and general cooking (it withstands high temperatures without burning) and add the seeds to salads, granola, and hummus.

DETOX BENEFITS
- ◆ Strong antioxidant activity
- ◆ Maintains balanced cholesterol levels

LEVEL III: CRUCIFEROUS VEGETABLES

Stimulate the liver's detox enzymes ◆ Help prevent cancer

◆ Increase levels of cleansing glutathione

BROCCOLI

Highly rated by the National Cancer Institute,

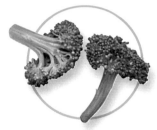

broccoli is a rich source of indole-3 carbinol, a compound that turns hormones into anticancer compounds. Broccoli increases levels of glutathione, a key antioxidant that helps the liver excrete toxic chemicals. It also contains sulforaphane, a potent phytonutrient that stimulates liver phase II detox enzymes (*see page 54*) and deactivates cancer cells. Also try sprouted broccoli seeds, which have 50 to 100 times more anticancer compounds than the vegetable.

BRUSSELS SPROUTS

The distinctive taste of brussels sprouts is the result of their high levels of sulfur-containing amino acids, such as cysteine and methionine, and the isothiocyanate sinigrin. Studies show that the latter kills precancerous cells. This effect is so powerful that even eating brussels sprouts only once in a while may destroy

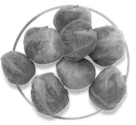

precancerous cells in the colon. Brussel sprouts are important vegetables at level III because they act to increase the body's levels of glutathione, an antioxidant that helps the liver dispose of toxins.

CABBAGE

Cabbage is a potent detoxifier at level III. It is a source of glucosinolate-derived chemicals called indoles, which help fight cancer. Numerous studies

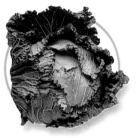

have linked diets rich in cabbage and other cruciferous vegetables with a reduced risk of cancer. Indoles and the flavonoids and carbinols in cabbage block cancer-causing agents by stimulating the liver's phase I and phase II detox enzymes (*see page 54*). Finally, cabbage raises the body's production of gluthathione, which is needed by the liver to excrete toxins such as exhaust fumes and drugs.

LEVEL III: LIVER SUPERFOODS

Aid liver function ◆ Eliminate toxic fats and free radicals

◆ Facilitate the digestion of fats

GLOBE ARTICHOKE

The globe artichoke is a renowned liver tonic that increases detoxification and the production of

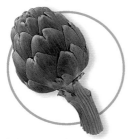

bile. Its purifying and protective effects make it a superb choice for detoxing the liver and easing liver ailments and its juice is a key remedy when the liver needs to be regenerated. The phytochemical cynarine helps in the excretion of bile and research shows that other constituents in the artichoke lower cholesterol levels and improve the metabolic assimilation of fats. The artichoke's diuretic action has a detoxifying effect on the kidneys.

DETOX BENEFITS
◆ Purifies and protects the liver
◆ Has a diuretic effect on the kidneys

AVOCADO

The avocado is a rich source of glutathione, which helps clear the body of harmful (oxidized) fats. The liver and kidneys need a high level of glutathione because of their involvement in phase II detox of drugs, chemicals, and environmental toxins (*see page 54*). The antioxidants in avocados encourage the elimination of toxic free radicals. Avocados

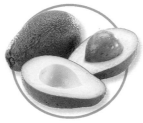

are a rich source of monounsaturated fat (oleic acid) and lecithin, which help digest fat in food, and in this way benefit those who have trouble digesting fats.

DETOX BENEFITS
◆ Helps clear body of harmful fats
◆ Antioxidants help eliminate toxic free radicals

BEETS

Beets have a regulating effect on the digestive system. They stimulate and strengthen the bowels, thus moving

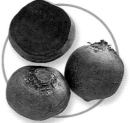

toxins out of the system. They also support kidney and liver function. Beets contain betaine, which aids fat metabolism by converting cholesterol into bile salts. Rich in potassium, fresh raw beet juice is a powerful blood cleanser and tonic. Furthermore, this vegetable can increase the uptake of oxygen in the cells by up to 400 percent and its red-colored constituents contain specific anticarcinogens.

DETOX BENEFITS
◆ Help the digestive system to work well
◆ Support liver and kidney function

LEVEL I: CULINARY HERBS & SPICES

Stimulate digestion ◆ Increase energy production

Antispasmodic properties ◆ Improve digestion

CARAWAY & DILL
Carum carvi &
Peucedanum graveolens
The seeds of these plants are useful at level I for relieving poor digestion. They ease symptoms such as colic, gas, hiccups, and abdominal bloating. Both seeds

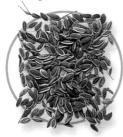

contain limonene, which can stimulate phase I and phase II detoxification enzymes (*see page 54*). They also aid the digestion of carbohydrates.

DETOX BENEFITS
◆ Reduce gas and abdominal bloating
◆ Contains limonene, which supports key detoxification enzymes

CORIANDER SEEDS
Coriandrum sativum
In Traditional Chinese Medicine (TCM) the "warming" action of the

seeds is considered to promote the circulation of *qi* (energy) in the stomach. They can help

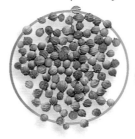

the body to digest carbohydrates and their antispasmodic properties make them helpful for relieving bloating and gas.

DETOX BENEFITS
◆ Facilitate digestion of carbohydrates
◆ Ease indigestion, bloating, and gas

GINGER
Zingiber officinale
This stimulating herb is essential for your level I detox. One of the best spices for improving digestion, it relieves colic, abdominal bloating, nausea, and diarrhea. Ginger stimulates digestive fire and is thought to increase the body's production of energy and raise its

metabolic rate. A strong cup of ginger tea half an hour before a meal can help stimulate digestive secretions, thereby aiding efficient digestion.

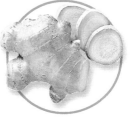

DETOX BENEFITS
◆ Improves the body's digestive processes
◆ Relieves the pain of poor digestion

GINGER TEA
Grate a piece of fresh ginger root big enough to give 2 tablespoons of grated ginger. Place in a mug and pour in boiling water. Cover and set aside to infuse for about 10 minutes. Strain the tea before drinking it and add honey, if desired.

For an extra warming effect, add a little of the strained ginger to the drink and chew it.

LEVEL II: CULINARY HERBS & SPICES

Antimicrobial and antifungal

Support immune system ◆ Alleviate viral infections

GARLIC
Allium sativum
Garlic is a major source of allylic sulfides, which are potent antioxidants that scavenge and destroy free radicals.

Garlic is effective at combatting a wide range of microbes, viruses,

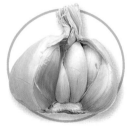

bacteria, parasites, and harmful fungi. Even when taken only in small doses, garlic is excellent at eliminating toxic microorganisms from the intestines. It is also a key level II detox herb because of its affinity with the Metal element in Traditional Chinese Medicine (TCM). Use garlic liberally in cooking throughout level II detox.

DETOX BENEFITS
- ◆ Powerful antioxidant and antimicrobial
- ◆ Supports the Metal element in TCM

OREGANO
Origanum vulgare
The active constituents in oregano (also known as wild marjoram) – thymol, carvacrol, and rosmarinic acid – account for its high antioxidant levels and potent antibacterial and antifungal properties. The herb is also a rich source of minerals, including calcium, magnesium, potassium, zinc, and iron. During

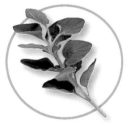

level II, include the fresh herb in side dishes as often as possible. You can also buy supplements containing wild oregano oil, which inhibits *Candida*: consult a herbalist about their use.

DETOX BENEFITS
- ◆ Destroys a wide range of detrimental viruses
- ◆ Rich source of minerals

THYME
Thymus vulgaris
In Traditional Chinese Medicine (TCM), thyme is considered to have important spiritual benefits. It revitalizes and uplifts the spirit. It also deepens the breathing and strengthens the

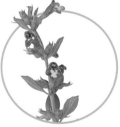

function of defensive *qi* (energy). On a physical level, thyme boosts the immune system and has expectorant properties, both of which make it ideal for clearing the lungs at level II. Use thyme liberally in cooking for its aromatic flavor.

In addition, herbalists recommend using a warm infusion of the herb to relieve constipation.

DETOX BENEFITS
- ◆ Decongests and cleanses the lungs
- ◆ Revitalizes and uplifts the spirit

LEVEL III: CULINARY HERBS & SPICES

Rich in antioxidants ◆ Stimulate bile production

Decongest and strengthen the liver ◆ Act as a diuretic

PARSLEY

Petroselinum crispum
This antioxidant herb contains iron, calcium, manganese, and vitamins A and C. Use it liberally in cooking at level III because it is rich in potassium and therefore is a diuretic, helping the kidneys to flush out toxins and acids in the urine. Parsley also

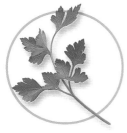

appears to strengthen the digestive organs, including the liver, perhaps because it contains the phyto-chemicals coumarins and limonene: the latter helps to support the liver's detoxification phases (*see page 54*).

DETOX BENEFITS
◆ Rich in potassium so a good diuretic
◆ Contains phyto-chemicals that aid detoxification

● **CAUTION**
Parsley is safe in cooking, but do not use the seeds in pregnancy or if your kidney is inflamed.

ROSEMARY

Rosmarinus officinalis
Include this herb in your diet at level III for its important antioxidants, which include carnosol, rosmanol, and limonene. Rosemary promotes liver and gallbladder function and stimulates production of bile, thus aiding fat digestion. As a diuretic,

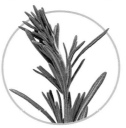

rosemary supports the kidneys, increasing the production of urine. In addition, the herb is believed to benefit the circulatory system.

DETOX BENEFITS
◆ Improves the digestion of fat
◆ Diuretic effect
◆ Strongly antioxidant

TURMERIC

Curcuma longa
The curcuminoids in turmeric are antioxidant and anti-inflammatory. The herb is used to decongest the liver,

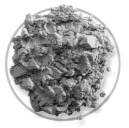

induce the flow of bile, dissolve gallstones, and strengthen the digestion. It strengthens the liver against toxins and free radicals and has been shown to inhibit chemically induced cell damage by an average of 75 percent. It also stimulates phase II liver detox (*see page 54*).

● **CAUTION**
Culinary quantities are safe but do not use medicinally if you have acute hepatitis, jaundice, or if you are pregnant.

DETOX BENEFITS
◆ Stimulates detox liver enzymes

HERBS & SUPPLEMENTS FOR LEVEL I

Alleviate allergic reactions ◆ Support digestion and nutrient absorption ◆ Increase energy ◆ Counter stress

BLUE-GREEN ALGAE

Blue-green algae nourishes the body at level I. It contain numerous antioxidants, vitamins, trace minerals, enzymes, and all eight amino acids in an easy-to-assimilate form. It

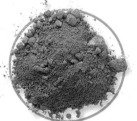

is alkaline-forming and can gently detoxify the body, helping eliminate the acidic by-products of stress. It can alleviate allergies by lowering elevated IgG levels (*see Glossary*), stabilize blood glucose fluctuations, and increase energy levels.

Dosage: 500–1,500 mg, twice a day (breakfast and midday meal)

DETOX BENEFITS
◆ Helps eliminate by-products of stress
◆ Can help to alleviate allergies

DIGESTIVE ENZYMES

People suffering from food allergies often have weak digestion and low levels of stomach acid. They may be helped by

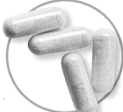

plant-derived digestive enzyme formulas, most of which are well tolerated by sensitive digestions. They contain a variety of enzymes – organic catalysts produced by living organisms that are necessary for the body's biochemical functions. These help the body break down proteins (protease), fats (lipase), as well as carbohydrates (amylase), thereby helping reestablish normal functioning of the digestive system.

Dosage: Formulas vary, so follow manufacturers' recommendations; take with each meal.

DETOX BENEFITS
◆ Assist the body in the digestion of food
◆ Enhance proper absorption of nutrients

KOREAN GINSENG

Panax ginseng
Ginseng is an adaptogenic plant, so-called because it has the ability to help the body adapt to the pressures of

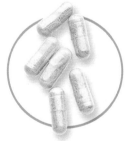

stress that weaken the adrenal glands. It has a reputation for enhancing stamina, energy, and vitality, and can be helpful at level I because it gives the body an extra boost while it is undergoing change.

Korean or Chinese ginseng is a powerful energy tonic, stronger than either American or Siberian ginseng, and must be taken with care.

American ginseng is milder and better for people under 50.

It is recommended that ginseng is not taken in the latter part of the day and that it is taken for a two-week period only, followed by two weeks off.

Dosage: 250 mg standardized extract, once or twice a day (breakfast and lunch)

DETOX BENEFITS
- Helps body adapt to pressures of stress
- Supports body during change

● **CAUTION**
Do not take ginseng during pregnancy. Avoid it also if you suffer from high blood pressure, palpitations, anxiety, or manic depressive disorder, or are taking steroids, caffeine, or blood-thinning medication.

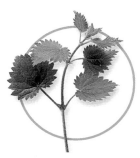

NETTLE
Urtica dioica
A very nutritious, chlorophyll-rich plant, nettle is a source of numerous nutrients, including silica, zinc, iron, vitamins B_2 and B_5, and folic acid. Because it supports the adrenal glands, the plant has incredible restorative and tonic properties. It is also an excellent blood purifier. Nettle has anti-inflammatory properties and, being a rich source of quercetin, can help reduce the incidence of allergic reactions.

Dosage: 200–300 mg of standardized extract, two to three times a day

DETOX BENEFITS
- Reduces incidence of allergic reactions
- Restorative, purifying, and tonic properties

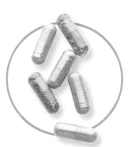

QUERCETIN
Quercetin, a bioflavonoid found in onions and nettles, is also available in supplement form. It reduces the intensity of allergic reactions by inhibiting the release of histamine and other inflammatory chemicals. It helps the intestinal wall to heal if damage has been caused by excessively permeable intestines or inflamed tissue. If left unchecked, such damage can aggravate the cycle of food allergies, creating further inflammation.

Dosage: 250–500 mg, twice a day

DETOX BENEFITS
- Reduces intensity of allergic reactions
- Anti-inflammatory and helps heal intestinal wall

PEPPERMINT
Mentha x piperita
Mint contains several essential oils, including

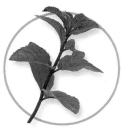

menthol, and works very effectively in the digestive tract, making it a key herb to include in level I. Its antispasmodic properties ease the pains caused by poor digestion: drink a cup of peppermint tea (made with dried or fresh herb) to help reduce symptoms of indigestion.

Dosage: 200 mg, usually once a day. Can be taken after meals if indigestion is a problem

DETOX BENEFITS
- Aids digestion
- Antispasmodic

HERBS & SUPPLEMENTS FOR LEVEL II

Cleanse the bowel ◆ Stimulate immune system

◆ Destroy harmful fungi, bacteria, and viruses

ASTRAGALUS

Astragalus membranaceus
This Chinese adaptogenic (antistress) herb helps alleviate fatigue by

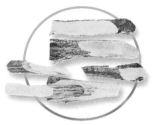

increasing energy production in the cells of the body. Astragalus has superior antiviral properties and helps restore the immune system. It increases the production of interferon and white blood cells and at the same time stimulates production of lymphocytes and antibodies. In this way it intensifies the body's ability to fight viruses and infections. Astragalus is also known for its ability to strengthen the lungs and to increase the rate of perspiration, which speeds the excretion of toxins.

Dosage: 200–300 mg standardized extract three times a day

DETOX BENEFITS
- ◆ Increases energy production
- ◆ Restores immune system

GOLDENSEAL

Hydrastis canadensis
Goldenseal is a key herb at level II because it has powerful antifungal properties and stimulates the immune system. One of its main active constituents, berberine, is a potent immune booster with a strong antibacterial action.

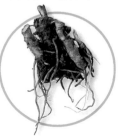

Berberine is known to kill harmful bacteria without disturbing the beneficial bacteria in the colon. When used to combat fungal infections, goldenseal can reduce the side effects that occur when the *Candida* overgrowth is killed. The herb also helps regulate bowel function.

Dosage: 400–1000 mg standardized extract twice a day

DETOX BENEFITS
- ◆ Kills harmful bacteria
- ◆ Effective against *Candida*

● **CAUTION**
Do not take this herb if pregnant.

ECHINACEA

Echinacea purpurea
Echinacea is an anti-inflammatory herb. It also increases the activity of the immune system, thus reinforcing the body's defense mechanism and speeding up recovery from infections such as colds and flu. Research has shown that echinacea inhibits viruses and helps destroy fungal infections such as *Candida*. Trials indicate that echinacea is more potent when taken intensively in the early stages of infection and over a two-week period without a break. The herb is also a source of fructo-oligosaccharides (FOS), a form of fiber that feeds the beneficial bacteria in the intestines.

Dosage: 300–500 mg standardized extract, 2–3 times a day, ideally for a two-week period

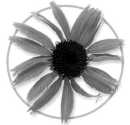

DETOX BENEFITS

- ◆ Enhances immunity and recovery from infections
- ◆ Fights viral, fungal, and bacterial infections

OLIVE LEAF
Olea europaea
This natural antibiotic has many phytochemicals that help destroy fungi, viruses, bacteria, and parasites, making it essential for level II detox. Containing

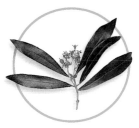

phenolic compounds, with powerful anti-oxidant properties, and oleuropein, which inhibits many harmful bacteria and intestinal parasites, it is effective in fighting infections, eliminating fungal or parasitic infest-ation, and supporting the immune system.

Dosage: 225–750 mg standardized extract, three times a day (between meals)

DETOX BENEFITS

- ◆ Powerful antioxidant
- ◆ Helps eliminate intestinal parasites

PAU D'ARCO
Tabebuia spp.
An ancient Incan herb, pau d'arco is the inner bark of the Brazilian "Tree of Life." It is a highly effective anti-microbial herb that strengthens the immune and lymphatic systems. One of its constituents, lapachol, has been shown to counteract certain parasites and its strong antifungal and anti-bacterial activity make it useful against *Candida*.

Dosage: 50–500 mg, twice a day

DETOX BENEFITS

- ◆ Antimicrobial and antifungal properties
- ◆ Supports lymphatic function

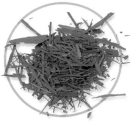

PSYLLIUM HUSKS
Plantago spp.
Psyllium husks are often used in bowel medicines since they possess mild laxative properties. They not only enlarge and soften bowel content, but also make it more slippery.

Psyllium husks contain both soluble and insoluble fiber, which are useful in cleansing the intestines in level II detox. The insoluble fiber is excellent for loosening old matter and increasing the size of the bulky mass traveling through the intestine. The gel-forming soluble fiber portion of psyllium can absorb toxins in the bowel and may also reduce the irritating effect of allergens associated with leaky gut syndrome.

Psyllium has also been known to relieve diarrhea and constipation, both

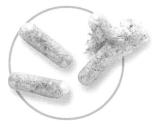

of which, if not corrected, can result in problems with the intestinal wall.

Dosage: 1,000–3,000 mg, one to three times a day, not with food and consumed with at least 10–17 fl.oz water

DETOX BENEFITS

- ◆ Soften bowel contents
- ◆ Laxative action, which helps to cleanse the bowel

HERBS & SUPPLEMENTS FOR LEVEL III

Help eliminate environmental toxins ◆ Soothe digestive problems ◆ Regenerate liver cells

MILK THISTLE

Silybum marianum
Silymarin, the active compound contained in this antioxidant herb, is one of the most potent liver-protective substances known. It has been shown to prevent and even reverse liver damage caused by environmental toxins, free radicals, drugs, alcohol, and chemicals in the diet. Silymarin stimulates protein synthesis, and also helps

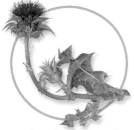

repair and regenerate the liver by encouraging the replacement of damaged liver cells with healthy ones. It boosts glutathione (*see opposite*) levels in the liver, which enhances the detoxification process.

Milk thistle has been shown to accelerate recovery time from the unpleasant side effects of chemotherapy due to its supportive action on the liver. The herb is also suggested to help treat depression and melancholy (considered in Traditional Chinese Medicine to be a form of liver stagnation or "anger turned in on the self").

Dosage: 120–160 mg three times a day

> DETOX BENEFITS
> ◆ Prevents and reverses liver damage
> ◆ Increases detoxifying glutathione

CHAMOMILE

Chamomilla recutita
According to Traditional Chinese Medicine (TCM), chamomile is a relaxing herb that soothes and cools the

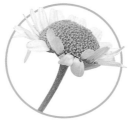

liver, which makes it useful for level III of the detox programme. It can also ease difficult digestion and relieve nausea. Chamomile is a traditional remedy for digestive disturbances.

Dosage: 250–1,000 mg standardized extract a day, between meals

> DETOX BENEFITS
> ◆ Soothes and cools the liver
> ◆ Reduces digestive disturbances

DANDELION

Taraxacum officinale
This common weed supports detoxification and is frequently recommended to help with liver toxicity and gallbladder complaints.

Dandelion increases the flow of bile and stimulates contraction of the gallbladder to release stored bile into the intestines. This aids in the breakdown of dietary fats, helps to prevent constipation, and may

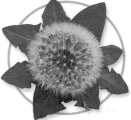

lead to a reduction in the incidence of gallstones. Its rich levels of minerals and potassium make dandelion a highly effective diuretic.

Dosage: 500–1,000 mg three times a day

> ### DETOX BENEFITS
> ◆ Stimulates contraction of gallbladder
> ◆ Useful cleansing and diuretic properties

SCHISANDRA

Schisandra chinensis
A powerful liver protector, schisandra also stimulates the immune and nervous systems. It is known as an adaptogenic herb because it has the ability to help the body adapt to the pressures of stress that would otherwise weaken the adrenal glands. Research

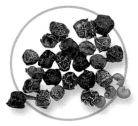

highlights the benefits of the active compounds schisandrins, which stimulate liver repair, prevent further liver damage, and also help to normalize the functioning of the liver.

Dosage: 200–400 mg twice a day

> ### DETOX BENEFITS
> ◆ Protects liver and helps it repair itself and function well
> ◆ Helps body adapt to change

GLUTATHIONE

Glutathione is the most important antioxidant produced naturally by the body's cells and it is also available as a supplement. It is made by combining three amino acids – cysteine, glutamic acid, and glycine.

The liver and kidneys have a high demand for

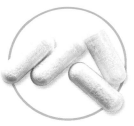

glutathione because they are involved in the level III detox processes that support the elimination of drugs, chemicals, and environmental toxins from the body. In addition to protecting cells from free-radical damage, glutathione helps eliminate alcohol, heavy metals, and pesticides. It does this by attaching itself to toxic compounds to neutralize their toxicity, so that the body can then excrete them safely.

Dosage: 250–500 mg twice a day, but not with food

> ### DETOX BENEFITS
> ◆ Protects cells from free radical damage
> ◆ Neutralizes toxicity of toxic compounds

LICORICE

Glycyrrhiza glabra
TCM believes licorice to have an affinity with the liver. It is thought to be able to harmonize and balance liver *qi* (energy).

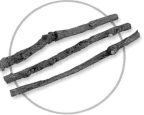

Scientific evidence has shown licorice has liver-supportive attributes that may justify its use as a powerful detoxifier. Often added in TCM to flavor and balance a formula, it is commonly used in its deglycyrrhized form (glycyrrhetinic acid taken out) in order to avoid the risk of swelling or high blood pressure that may be associated with long-term use of standard licorice root.

Dosage: 500–1,500 mg standardized extract a day, between meals

> ### DETOX BENEFITS
> ◆ Powerful detoxifying agent
> ◆ Harmonizes and balances liver *qi* (energy)

SPA TECHNIQUES FOR LEVEL I

Support the body during detoxification ◆

Boost energy levels ◆ Relieve digestive complaints

REFLEXOLOGY

At level I, focus on the reflex zones described below (*see also chart, page 121*) to gently support and stimulate digestion. Using the technique on page 30, massage the zones when they feel congested, every few days.

First massage the zone for the spleen/pancreas, which is found on the left

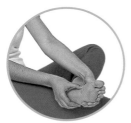

foot (*see picture above*). Then work on the reflex point for the stomach, located on the inner side of the left foot. Repeat on the right foot. Finally, massage the points for the adrenal glands, which sit above the kidney zones on both feet, and are often tender to touch.

● **CAUTION**
See pages 9 and 30.

ACUPRESSURE

The following acupoints are the primary pressure points for a level I detox.

Using your thumb, gently hold or massage each point several times a day for up to a minute several times a day.

● **CAUTION**
See pages 9 and 31.

SPLEEN 6

A valuable acupoint for many reasons, spleen 6 is especially useful; it is the crossing point of the spleen, liver, and kidney meridians (energy channels in Traditional Chinese Medicine: *see page 32*). It is thought, therefore, to have a beneficial impact on liver and kidney *qi* (energy), supporting and helping to increase it. Spleen 6

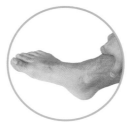

lies $1^1/_4$–$1^1/_2$ in (3–4 cm) above the inside of the ankle bone (*see picture above*) on both legs, and is often tender to touch.

● **CAUTION**
Do not use this acupoint during pregnancy.

STOMACH 36

This key acupoint helps support the whole body, strengthens digestion, and boosts energy levels. It is located on the outside of the shin on both legs,

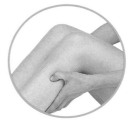

2 in (5 cm) beneath the outer part of the knee-bone (*see picture above*).

BLADDER 23

Massaging these points stimulates the kidney and adrenal glands and boosts energy levels. They lie on either side of the spine (*see picture below*), and are stimulated by putting your hands on your hips and using your thumbs to press on the points. In

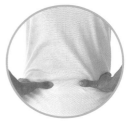

Traditional Chinese Medicine it is important to protect this region, and in Japan, a *harikame* (a band around the kidney and navel area) is worn to keep the body healthy and the immune system strong. To restore your energy levels using this approach, tie a scarf around your waist to cover an area 6¹/₂ in (16 cm) wide at the back and 3¹/₂ in (8 cm) deep above and below the waist.

AROMATHERAPY

Aromatherapists believe that massaging essential oils into the skin benefits the digestive system and eases symptoms such as bloating and indigestion.

This is best done when you can relax, later in the day. Make a massage oil blend using essential oils (*see page 29*). Apply to your abdomen, focusing on the left-hand side of your rib cage, where your spleen and stomach are located. Also apply the oil to the reflex points on your feet and the relevant acupressure points.

● **CAUTION**
See pages 9 and 29.

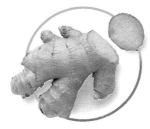

GINGER OIL
Ginger possesses drying, warming, and stimulating properties. It is used to strengthen the digestive system, increase energy levels, and ease symptoms such as nausea, abdominal distension, poor appetite, and fatigue.

On an emotional level it may help to activate and fire the willpower, so it is ideal if apathy or procrastination strike at the beginning of this program, possibly helping encourage you to keep your resolve.

LEMON OIL
Yellow is associated with the Earth element and digestion in Traditional Chinese Medicine. Lemon essential oil supports the

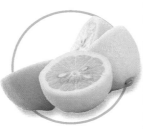

function of the spleen, which is to transform food into energy that can be circulated around the body by the blood. Lemon oil may help reduce lymphatic congestion and obesity, which can be a result of poor digestion. An uplifting oil to inhale, it stimulates the liver and the pancreas, the organ involved in keeping blood glucose levels stable.

FENNEL OIL
Useful for clearing excess weight and congestion, this mildly diuretic oil stimulates the lymphatic system. It is thought to regulate appetite levels and reduce the appetite when overindulging. A *yang* tonic in Traditional Chinese Medicine, it is

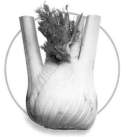

energy-giving, since it increases both spleen and adrenal *qi* (energy), two areas of the body being fortified in level I. Fennel oil is often used to reduce abdominal pain and gas caused by poor digestion and food intolerance.

SKIN-BRUSHING
The lymphatic system can easily become sluggish; skin-brushing can help improve circulation and enhance skin texture. Use a long-handled, natural-bristle brush on dry skin for 2–3 minutes before taking a shower, following the sequence below:
◆ Brush the soles and tops of the feet, and up the legs.
◆ Sweep toward the heart and over the upper breast, aiming for the armpit, to assist lymph drainage.
◆ Raise each arm and gently brush from the hand down to the armpit.
◆ Sweep from the buttocks up the back to the neck.
◆ Brush up the inside of the right hipbone, across beneath the ribs, and down the left side, making a circle that follows the direction of the colon.

SPA TECHNIQUES FOR LEVEL II

Encourage the body to "let go" ◆ Promote a feeling of

release ◆ Stimulate the organs of elimination

REFLEXOLOGY

In a level II detox you are working on the area of the foot that corresponds to the colon (*see chart, page 121*). Massage these reflex points when they feel congested, every few

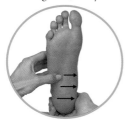

days, using the thumbing technique on page 30.

The colon has quite a complicated reflex zone. Starting on the left foot, working on the ileocecal valve and ascending colon, across half the transverse colon, and then continue onto your right foot. Still following the transverse colon across the foot, work your way down the descending colon, finishing at the rectum. Then massage the reflex for the small intestine, found on both feet. "Walk" your thumb in straight lines from the outer edge of the foot toward the inside edge (*see picture above*). Drink several glasses of water

after working on your intestines. If you suffer from excess mucus, massage the pads of the toes to help decongest and release your sinuses.

● **CAUTION**
See pages 9 and 30.

ACUPRESSURE

The main acupoints for level II are described below. Hold or massage each one several times a day as shown, pressing firmly for 1–2 minutes.

● **CAUTION**
See pages 9 and 31.

LARGE INTESTINE 4

This acupoint is used to support detoxification

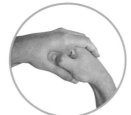

and elimination by improving the function of the large intestine. If you have constipation, the point may feel congested and painful. The point lies on the webbed section of either hand, between the thumb and first finger (*see picture above*).

LARGE INTESTINE 11

Good for constipation, Large Intestine 11 is used to stimulate the bowel. When combined with Large Intestine 4 (LI 4), it is believed to have the additional benefit of helping to improve the complexion. Like LI 4, it often feels a little sore.

To find this acupoint, which is located on both arms, bend your elbow and take the thumb of

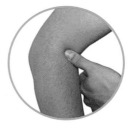

the other hand along the crease until you can feel an indentation before the bone (*see picture above*).

LUNG 7

Used to strengthen the respiratory system, Lung 7 is a good preventive point to massage when you want to support the lungs and enhance their ability to "let go of the old" and to circulate oxygen around the body. It is also a useful point to

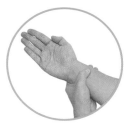

massage in the early stages of coughs, colds, and infections.

Lung 7 is 1 in (2.5 cm) from the wrist crease on the inside of both forearms, in line with the thumb (*see picture above*).

AROMATHERAPY

At level II, you can use essential oils to encourage detoxification, stimulate lymphatic drainage, strengthen the immune system (using *wei qi*, or defensive energy), and enhance breathing.

● CAUTION

For general cautions, see pages 9 and 29.

TEA TREE OIL

This natural antibiotic has powerful antifungal and antiviral properties. Aromatherapists use the essential oil for problems such as *Candida* and yeast infections; tea tree pessaries are a natural alternative to conventional versions for easing the irritation of yeast infections. In TCM, tea

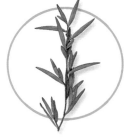

tree oil is used to increase resistance to infection. It is believed to strengthen the protective *wei qi*, or defensive energy, in the body and thus support the immune system.

Aromatherapists use the diluted oil to treat many fungal and bacterial infections. Do a patch test first; it can irritate the skin. Use the diluted oil (*see page 29*), daily or as required, to massage the chest, or apply it to the relevant reflex and acupressure points.

● CAUTION

May cause skin irritation.

EUCALYPTUS OIL

Antibacterial and anti-viral, this oil has a strong affinity with the immune and respiratory systems. On a psychological level,

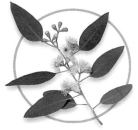

it is uplifting and helps to release negative feelings or grief, allowing you to let go of the past and open your mind to new ideas.

Massage the diluted oil (*see page 29*) onto the chest, or apply the oil to the relevant reflex and acupressure points. You could also add 3 drops of oil to a basin of steaming hot water and inhale for 10 minutes with a towel over your head. Repeat daily or when congested.

FRANKINCENSE OIL

This oil is known for its capacity to strengthen the body's physical defense system and rebuild energy levels when the immune system is weak. Revered as an herb of protection in TCM, frankincense is

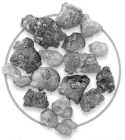

said to strengthen spiritual defenses when *wei qi* (defensive energy) is low and you are susceptible to negative energies. Used to calm and to encourage a deeper level of breathing, helping you let go of emotions and stale air, it is ideal to inhale before or during meditation. To do this, add 4 drops of undiluted oil to an aromatherapy burner and inhale while practicing deep breathing or meditation.

SKIN-BRUSHING

At level I, this is done on dry skin before a shower. At level II, follow the skin-brushing sequence (*see page 81*) with a warm shower, then switch to a cold shower to dilate and contract the blood vessels and stimulate activity in the lymphatic system.

Don't be alarmed to see mucus in stools after skin-brushing: this shows that the body is clearing away old toxins.

SPA TECHNIQUES FOR LEVEL III

Dissolve further toxins ◆ Promote a deeper level of purification ◆ Create a state of inner calm

REFLEXOLOGY

At level III, the focus is on the liver, gallbladder, and kidneys. Massage these reflexes (*see chart, page 121*) every few days, or when they feel congested.

First, gently massage the liver reflex situated on the right foot, and the gallbladder reflex, which is just below the liver reflex, for a minute. To help the kidneys filter toxins more effectively, massage the

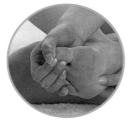

bladder reflexes, located on the inside of both feet near the heel. Starting on the bladder point, "walk" your thumb, tracing along the tendon (which represents the urethra) until you reach the kidney point (*see picture above*). Massage this point to loosen any "crystals" that may have accumulated. According to reflexology theory (*see page 30*), the liver rules the eyes, so massage the eye reflex points on both feet as a preventive technique and to strengthen vision. Drink plenty of water after working these areas.
● **CAUTION**
See pages 9 and 30.

ACUPRESSURE

The focus in acupressure at level III is supporting and decongesting the liver and gallbladder. To do this, hold or massage the following acupoints firmly as shown for 1–2 minutes **twice** a day.
● **CAUTION**
See pages 9 and 31.

LIVER 3

A highly significant point on the body, the liver is often overworked and abused. Liver 3 is used to strengthen the liver, calm the nervous system, and support the immune system. Massaging it for 1–2 minutes may relieve toxic headaches, reduce allergic sensitivity, and

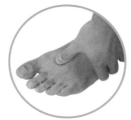

help overcome the effects of stress or toxins in the body. On both feet, find the point between the first and second toes, about 1 in (2.5 cm) away from the base of the toes (*see picture, below left*).

GALLBLADDER 20

Massage this point if you have headaches while detoxifying. It improves circulation to the facial area and relieves tension in the head and neck. Any congestion in the body makes this point sore to touch, so gently massage along the base of the skull, too. Gallbladder 20 lies at the base of the

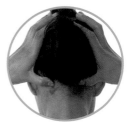

skull between the neck muscles of the spine (*see picture above*).

GALLBLADDER 21

Find the acupoint at that painful area at the top of the shoulders, on the muscle at the base of the neck (*see picture below*). This is a classic area for reflecting a state of tension and disharmony. Massaging both points on either shoulder may help

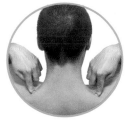

fatigue and also relieves pain and stiffness in the shoulders and upper back.

AROMATHERAPY

According to Traditional Chinese Medicine (TCM), these three essential oils harmonize and unblock liver *qi* (energy) to allow an even flow of energy around the body. Specific oils are used to cool an overheated and abused liver and support detox on a deeper level.

● CAUTION

For general cautions, see pages 9 and 29.

MANDARIN OIL

In TCM, this essential oil has a stimulant effect on both the gallbladder and the liver. It is used to help release liver stagnation, which upsets the flow of *qi* (energy) and blood, leading to problems such

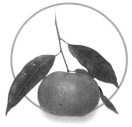

as abdominal distension, indigestion, nauseous headaches, menstrual disorders, muscle stiffness, emotional frustration, mood swings, and anger. By encouraging bile secretion, the oil helps the body break down fats more efficiently. Apply in dilution (*see page 29*) to the right-hand side of the rib cage, where your liver and gallbladder lie and to the lower back, where your kidneys are located. You can also apply the oil to the relevant reflex and acupressure points.

ROSEMARY OIL

A stimulating tonic oil in TCM, rosemary is held to increase the circulation of

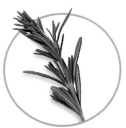

blood and *qi* (energy) in the body, boosting energy levels. Long known as a mentally invigorating oil, it is said to enhance the cellular uptake of oxygen. New research also suggests that it possesses powerful antioxidant properties. By stimulating bile flow, the oil aids the digestion and the assimilation of fats, and may help to alleviate allergies. Use in dilution (*see page 29*), applying to the right-hand side of the rib cage, where your liver and gallbladder lie, and to the lower back, where

your kidneys are located. You can also apply the oil to the relevant reflex and acupressure points.

● CAUTION

Do not use this oil during pregnancy or if you have epilepsy. Always use in a diluted solution.

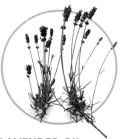

LAVENDER OIL

A safe and soothing oil, lavender possesses nerve-relaxant properties and is valued in TCM to help release liver stagnation. Its cooling properties are thought to clear latent heat that can build up in the liver, generating further stagnation. This oil promotes deep, sound sleep and diffuses over-heated emotions such as anger and rage, creating inner peace. Massage the temples with diluted oil (*see page 29*) when you are tense or have a headache.

SKIN-BRUSHING

Skin-brushing makes the skin stronger, so apply firmer pressure at level III, still using the sequence on page 81. As you brush, visualize your body being cleansed and purified, and see toxins being dredged into the lymphatic system. The body may get used to skin-brushing after time; if so, reduce the frequency to just twice a week.

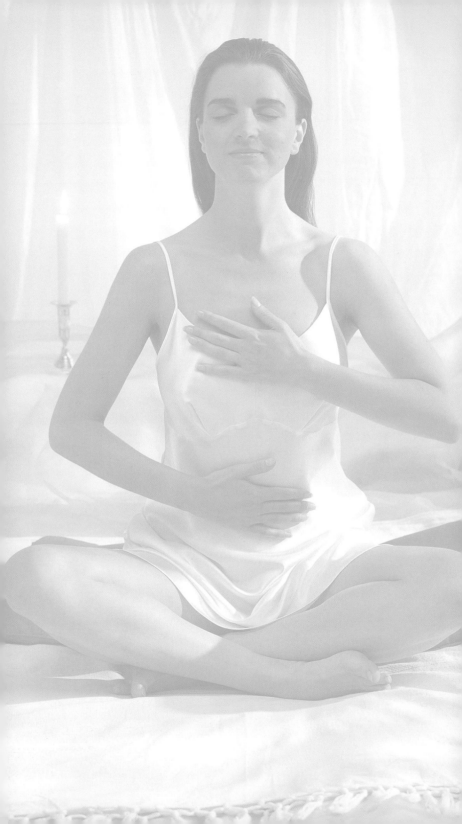

MIND DETOX

"I AM NOW COMPLETELY RELAXED IN BODY AND MIND. I AM RECEPTIVE TO NATURE'S HARMONIOUS AND INVIGORATING VIBRATIONS – THEY DISPEL THE DISCORDANT AND DESTRUCTIVE VIBRATIONS OF HURRY, WORRY, FEAR, AND ANGER. NEW LIFE, NEW HEALTH, NEW STRENGTH ARE ENTERING INTO ME WITH EVERY BREATH, PERVADING MY WHOLE BEING."

AFFIRMATION BY HENRY LINDLAHR

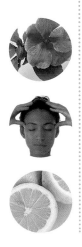

DETOXING THE MIND & EMOTIONS

Mental detoxification cleanses the mind of negative thought patterns and uncovers hidden emotions such as grief, anger, or fear, transforming them into feelings of forgiveness, hope, love, and joy.

MIND-BODY CONNECTION

Conventional Western medicine now recognizes (as Eastern systems of healing have for centuries) that health and disease are related not only to the chemical condition of the cells and physiology of the body, but also to a person's state of mind. Research has shown that the cells that carry emotions to the brain are also present in the immune system and that the molecular messengers of the cells connect the body's immune, nervous, and endocrine systems. What we think and feel – our emotional state of health – does indeed have an impact on the whole immune system and thus has a profound effect on health.

This is why the creation of a positive emotional attitude is an essential part of a successful detox and healing program. Dealing with negative emotional patterns can help us to acknowledge and let go of problems from the past, such as unhappy childhood experiences or difficult relationships.

NATUROPATHIC MEDICINE

Practitioners of naturopathy believe that a variety of factors contribute toward the health of body and mind. The internal and external factors that can have an influence on the body's health and on mental and spiritual well-being are highlighted, right.

Diet
Nutrition through food and drink

Lifestyle
Social habits, stresses of daily life

Body
Exercise, physical healing therapies

Environment
Living and work spaces, quality of air, sunlight

Spiritual
Meditation and contemplation

Heredity
Genetic inheritance

Mind
Positive and negative thoughts

EMOTIONS AND FIVE ELEMENTS

Traditional Chinese Medicine (TCM) recognizes a connection between the emotions and the health of the body. The five primary emotions connected to the five elements of TCM philosophy are shown, right.

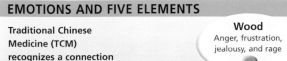

Wood
Anger, frustration, jealousy, and rage

Water
Fear and shock

Fire
Laughter, love, and joy

Metal
Grief and an inability to let go

Earth
Obsession, worry, and a need for sympathy

THE NATUROPATHIC APPROACH

A holistic approach to health, such as that of naturopathy, recognizes the significance of the interconnection of mind, body, and spirit. Naturopaths believe that a variety of factors, both within the body and outside it, contribute toward disease or health (*see box opposite*). For detox to be successful, all of these factors must be addressed.

Far from being a "new-age" idea, this philosophy dates back centuries. For example, Dr. Henry Lindlahr MD, the pioneering US naturopath, focused on the physical aspects of naturopathy such as detox, massage, spinal manipulation, and diet. However, he also embraced the psychological and spiritual aspects, recognizing that negative thoughts have a detrimental effect on the body's innate life force.

THE EASTERN APPROACH

In Traditional Chinese Medicine (TCM), emotional distress is held to compromise health, especially when emotions are particularly intense or have been suppressed. TCM connects five main emotions to the five elements (*see box above*).

Worry or a need for sympathy are the primary emotions associated with the Earth element (which is addressed at level I): a constant need for sympathy, incessant fretting, hypochondriac tendencies and obsessional behavior patterns are all common indicators. Conversely, an aversion to these traits and a dislike of being fussed over may also indicate the Earth element.

Fear and shock are the primary emotions tied to the kidneys and the Water element. These natural emotions can deplete us when prolonged. The emotions of grief and not being able to let go of the past are linked to the Metal element (addressed at level II).

Excessive jealousy, irritation, anger, or suppressed rage point to the Wood element (worked on at level III). Laughter, love, and joy are connected to the heart and are Fire element emotions; an imbalance can manifest in an inability to laugh or demonstrate love.

PROGRAM FOR LEVEL I

This first-level mind-detox plan focuses on nourishing the self. It involves getting rid of emotional crutches, especially food, that may have developed over the years to support flagging self-confidence and build self-esteem.

AIMS OF THE PROGRAM

The aim of this mind detox program is to help you establish a good relationship with yourself and develop a true sense of who you are. If you feel you are failing to reach your goals, this may help you to understand why. A lack of self-nourishment and loss of self-esteem can result in self-destructive behavior, including an obsessive attitude toward food, which may result in eating disorders such as

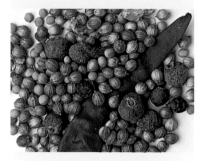

overeating and deprivation regimes. The level I mind detox aims to help you throw away emotional crutches like food and find time to nourish yourself in body and mind.

Your Program

- Be positive. Do not put off taking your first step on this self-nourishing program.

- Rethink your cooking and eating habits (*see opposite*).

- Start each day with an affirmation to nourish the emotions (*see page 92*).

- Before the first meal of the day, practice the Breath of Life (*see page 100*) to help keep you focused and calm.

- Meditate for 15 minutes a day (*see pages 108–109*) to help develop inner strength.

- For advice on how long to stay at level I, see page 20.

Food and the Emotions

As you begin to treat yourself with more care and respect, you will gravitate toward supportive and nourishing foods. But you still might find yourself using food as a substitute for affection and love, especially when feeling stressed. The taste associated with the Earth element in Traditional Chinese Medicine is sweetness, and eating candy in excess is a way of giving yourself the sweetness that you may feel nobody else is giving you. It also connects to the use of candy as a reward in childhood. Do not be disappointed if, during your work on this program, you devour the contents of the cookie jar. This is normal: you cannot achieve perfection overnight.

Detoxing the Kitchen

An essential step to success in level I is ruthlessly to clear your kitchen of the high-fat, high-sugar, nutritionally unsound comfort foods that have been sustaining you for far too long. Use the ideas below to plan a new eating program that enables your body to reach its optimum level.

New Eating Habits

◆ Set aside a day to go through your kitchen cabinets and throw out all the processed and refined foods you find there.

◆ Take this handbook out on a shopping trip. Choose foods and ingredients from level I of the body detox program and catalog (see *pages 38–39 and 59–61*) to restock your kitchen. Where possible, select locally grown fruits and vegetables which are fresher, retain more nutrients, and keep your body more in tune with the seasons than foods that have had to travel some distance.

◆ Once you have the right ingredients, make a pact with yourself to become more creative in the kitchen. Try out new recipes, be experimental, and see how much more delicious and satisfying your meals become.

◆ Many of the foods suggested have a wonderful flavor but some of the grains can be a little bland. Do not reach for the salt shaker. Instead, use fresh garden herbs, lemons, and spices to flavor food. Allow your taste buds to adjust to these exciting new flavors.

◆ Use more warming spices – they not only help support digestion but can also be emotionally comforting; for example, simply adding turmeric to rice gives it a rich golden appearance that makes it so much more appetizing. In addition, the color yellow nurtures the Earth element in TCM and supports the digestion.

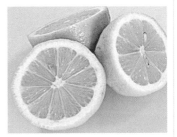

◆ Satisfy all your senses when you eat: first smell the food and feast your eyes on its visual appearance, then savor the taste and appreciate the contrasting textures. According to TCM, this increases the absorption of nutrients and enhances the digestive process.

◆ Be in a peaceful state of mind when you eat. This aids the digestion and assimilation of all the nutrients in the foods.

Understanding Problems

As you work through this level of mind detox, you will feel motivated and strong at times but vulnerable at others, and you may want to fall back on old, destructive habits. Be gentle and

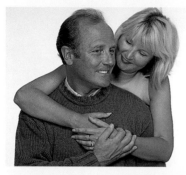

understanding with yourself, as working through this part of the reflective process is an essential aspect of the program.

◆ As the first step in the nurturing process, think about where your lack of self-love stems from and how it manifests in the old habits. Your beliefs about yourself will have been established in your formative years.

◆ Think about how relationships with your parents, siblings, and friends have had a profound effect on your self-image and ability to love yourself.

◆ Consider whether food became a way of filling an inner emptiness caused by a lack of affection and acceptance. Start to appreciate that only you can take steps towards improving your confidence and self-image.

Most importantly, never forget that self-love is a prerequisite to bringing about positive change in life. Awareness is not enough: you need to be fully committed to the idea of change.

An Eastern Perspective

In Traditional Chinese Medicine, nourishment, support, and self-care are the positive traits of a balanced, strong Earth element. The three levels of body, mind, and spirit detox in this program will help you balance these characteristics within yourself.

Symptoms of an unbalanced Earth element include worry, negativity, obsessional behavior, overdependency and an unfulfilled need for support. When you are worried, your stomach can feel tied up in knots and you feel nauseous, hence the expression "letting something gnaw away inside you."

However, developing a strong center by meditating (*see pages 108–109*), nurturing yourself, and learning to take advantage of every opportunity for laughter can encourage and support the healing process.

Affirmation

"I now make a commitment to respect, nurture, and care for my body. I will choose to nourish it with vital health-giving foods and support it with loving thoughts."

PROGRAM FOR LEVEL II

This program focuses on repairing and strengthening the immune system. It encourages you to let go of long-held, energy-sapping negative emotions that hinder personal growth and replace them with positive ideas.

AIMS OF THE PROGRAM

Research has shown that people who have a positive attitude to life get fewer viral infections and have stronger immune systems than those without. Low self-esteem, a problem tackled in the level I mind detox, is another potential contributory factor in the development of a weakened immune system. What you have gained from the level I mind-detox program – belief in yourself and responsibility for your emotional attitude – remains important at level II.

Level II teaches you to focus on positive, uplifting, nurturing thoughts and feelings and give less energy to negative thought patterns that destroy peace of mind and undermine health.

In this program it is important to acknowledge rather than suppress your emotions. Traditional Chinese Medicine teaches that all emotions, from joy to grief, must be expressed. Crying to release pain, for example, has a physiological

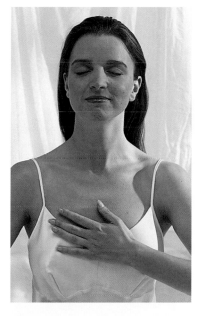

function – tears shed with emotion contain stress hormones and manganese (found in high concentrations in the brains of depressed people).

An aim of the level II plan is to encourage you to let go of emotional pain and to have the awareness and understanding that letting go is necessary for your psychological development and movement forward in life.

Your Program

♦ Continue the level I dietary program, adding items from the level II body-detox program and catalog (see pages 46–48 and 63–66).

♦ As you did in the kitchen at level I, clear the bathroom and bedroom of anything that may be harmful (see below right).

♦ Repeat constructive affirmations that urge "letting go" of the past (see opposite).

♦ Practice deep breathing (see page 100) for about 5 minutes daily to increase oxygen levels in the lungs and help rid them of stagnant carbon dioxide.

♦ Set aside time every day for the Protective and Letting Go meditations (see pages 110–11) to help you focus on nurturing, positive, and uplifting thoughts.

♦ For advice on how long to stay at level II, see page 20.

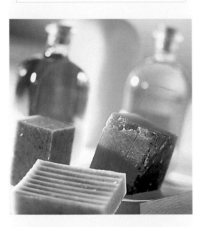

Bathroom and Bedroom Detox

Start your level II by getting rid of the many damaging toxins that modern manufacturing has allowed to creep into household and personal care products, from detergents to shampoos, lotions, and cosmetics.

When you apply these creams and potions to your skin, chemicals in the products may be absorbed into the blood in the same way that hormone replacement therapy and nicotine patches work. This may add to the body's toxic load, as can antiperspirants, which may contain potentially toxic metals such as aluminum. Use the ideas below to eliminate potentially toxic items from your bathroom and bedroom.

Toxin Clear-out

♦ Clear from the bathroom cabinet products that contain many chemicals.

♦ Visit a natural health store to stock up on natural or organic alternative products, such as deodorant stones made from crystals or soap containing essential oils instead of bath and shower gels based on petroleum. These support your health as well as animal welfare and the environment.

♦ Remove from your wardrobe clothes you haven't worn often or items that have any negative associations. Throw out or give away anything made with synthetic fabrics. Base your newly "detoxed" wardrobe on clothes made of natural fibers such as silk, wool, cotton, and linen. Be ruthless in this procedure: you will feel much lighter and clearer in mind once the clutter has been eliminated.

An Eastern Perspective

Conventional Western medicine views the lungs purely practically: they are organs that take in the oxygen necessary to sustain life and eliminate carbon dioxide and toxins. Traditional Chinese Medicine (TCM) gives the lungs a dual rhythmic function. The lungs receive the "heavenly *qi*" (energy) that gives a sense of meaning to life and allow the letting go of old emotions. Grief and loss can disrupt this function, and if the flow of energy is weak, apathy and a lack of inspiration can result.

In TCM the bodily soul, or *P'o*, is connected to the Metal element in the Five Elements table (*see page 33*) and is affected by negative emotions, including remorse and pessimism. This is why detoxification work on the lungs and the large intestine (Metal element organs of elimination) may cause grief and old hurts to surface.

The TCM body clock time for the lungs is 3–5am, a common time to wake with breathing difficulties or feelings of grief for a bereavement or loss. Intense grief can have a profound effect on health; not fully grieving may develop into a Metal element depression that manifests as an inability to progress forward in life. Equally, there comes a time to let go and move on. Use level II to resolve such issues.

The large intestine, the other Metal element organ, is involved in letting go of impurities. TCM considers constipation to be a condition in which the body physically and emotionally holds on to old stuff. This can reflect an inability to let go of the past and of negative thoughts. Use the level II mind detox to forgive and learn from experience. While doing the deep breathing, visualize letting go of grief, pain, and unhelpful past events.

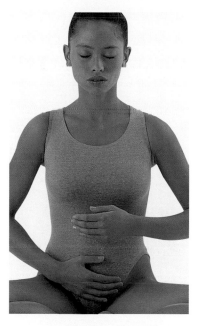

Affirmation

"It is safe to let go of anything that no longer nourishes my mind, body, and spirit. With every exhalation I release old pain, and every breath I draw in brings inspiration and protection."

PROGRAM FOR LEVEL III

Having successfully worked through levels I and II, you are now ready to move forward with your mind-detoxification program to a level that concentrates on planning positively for the future.

AIMS OF THE PROGRAM

Levels I and II of the mind-detox program were concerned with releasing accumulated negative emotions that have a detrimental effect on your immune system and with letting go of toxic thoughts. Now, with your psychological and physiological well-being enhanced, you can work more positively in level III, planning ahead for the future and starting afresh. Level III also aims to give your life a sense of calmness and endow you with the ability to flow and adapt to difficult situations with ease and understanding. Detoxing the liver, the main target of the level III body-detox program, is essential to a successful completion of this aim.

Making a New Beginning

Traditional Chinese Medicine (TCM) sees spring, associated with the Wood element in the Five Elements table (*see page 33*), as a time of new growth. For you,

Your Program
◆ Continue with your diet and eating plan, adding foods from the level III body-detox program and catalog (*see pages 54–58 and 67–70*).
◆ Start each day with a helpful affirmation (*see page 98*).
◆ Before breakfast, practice the Breath of Life (*see page 100*).
◆ Do 20–30 minutes of yoga or cardiovascular exercise 5 times a week (*see pages 116–17*).
◆ Do the level III meditations every day (*see pages 112–13*).
◆ Practice physically releasing pent-up feelings of frustration and anger (*see opposite*).
◆ For advice on how long to stay at level III, see page 21.

the start of nature's year is an ideal time to plant the seeds of the future and sow your plans, dreams, and aspirations.

The oak tree begins its journey as an acorn, a single shoot that pushes through the earth, flexible enough to work around any obstacles that could prevent its growth. Given the right nourishment,

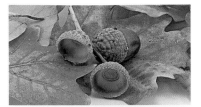

the acorn matures into a strong, beautiful oak tree. Just like the acorn, you will encounter many obstacles and challenges in life. How you respond emotionally to these makes a difference to your health and well-being. Often, when a course of action is blocked, frustration and irritation begin to build. The work you do to strengthen and decongest your liver in the level III body-detox program helps this sense of irritation to flow and adapt to situations instead of escalating to full-blown anger.

Releasing Emotions

Before the seeds of a new start can be sown, any suppressed emotions associated in TCM with an imbalanced liver must be safely detoxed. The liver is a powerful center for body detoxing and psychologically it can become the dumping ground for poisonous emotions that we feel unable to express: rage, envy, hatred, and self-disgust. Such feelings deplete energy levels and can weaken and impair liver function. Anger is the key emotion of the liver, which is why, when cleansing it at this

deep level, you may reexperience long-suppressed anger or depression ("anger turned inward"). While TCM believes that anger in short, explosive bursts is healthy, such behavior is not acceptable in our society. But coming to terms with anger and releasing it constructively is important in the healing process: below are some acceptable ways of doing this.

Expressing Anger

♦ When frustrations cause your mental energy to flag, find a quiet space where you will not be disturbed and physically get the anger out by punching a pillow and stamping your feet.

♦ Reenact in your quiet space the scenario that led to your frustration and anger. Imagine the situation and say exactly what you would have liked to have said at the time. This is a very powerful, emotion-releasing exercise.

♦ Another effective way to release frustration and anger is to write your feelings down in a letter (but do not send it).

♦ Freeing yourself of emotional pain is a priority in this stage of the detox. If your emotions are severely repressed and you are unable to get in touch with your anger, it may be useful to get the help of a psychotherapist.

♦ Once you feel you have released some inner anger, practice the affirmation on page 98 to help soothe and heal body, emotions, and soul.

An Eastern Perspective

In Traditional Chinese Medicine (TCM), the liver is the planner while its partner Wood element organ, the gallbladder, is the courageous decision-maker. Thus

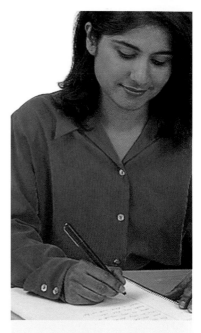

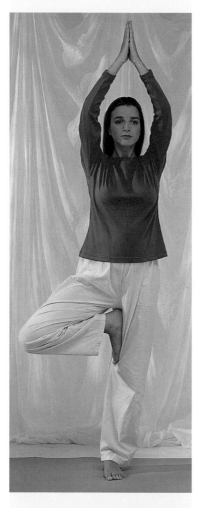

compassion, purpose, and vision; without these it is discontented and despairing. Alcohol, toxins, and strong emotions such as anger also upset it. Frustration and resentment can send it into a negative spiral, causing critical, intolerant behavior and a loss of aspiration and motivation.

Strengthening the liver sharpens your decision-making: now is the time to define your goals – with a detoxed liver you have a strong capacity to plan your life and its future direction.

indecisive, disorganized actions indicate an imbalance in the liver. In TCM, the spiritual soul, or *Hun*, lies in the liver, and thrives on guiding you through life with

Affirmation

"I have the courage to release toxic emotions in a positive and constructive manner. I possess the clarity of vision to renew and plan my future aspirations, so enabling me to move forward on my life's journey."

AFFIRMATIONS

Retrain the subconscious mind ◆ Harness the power of

positive thinking ◆ Exploit the mind-body connection

ANYWHERE, ANY TIME
Positive affirmations can be
made sitting quietly or
when you are on the move.

KEY PRINCIPLES

Eastern medicine, from Traditional Chinese Medicine to Indian Ayurveda, is holistic in that it addresses physical health and mental and spiritual well-being as a whole. It recognizes the significant impact that emotional imbalances or negative beliefs can have on the body's ability to heal itself. Hippocratic doctrine adhered to this belief until the 17th century. Then, conventional Western medicine adopted an analytical model, based on the Cartesian reductionist theory of René Descartes, which denied any influence of the mind on the body. Today, Western

medicine is returning to a pre-Cartesian view. Pioneering research has revealed evidence of a mind-body connection by showing that neuro-transmitters can transform thoughts and emotions into clear physiological changes. Affirmations exploit this process. They are short positive statements of intent such as, "I am loved." Repeating them is said to retrain the subconscious mind to avoid habitual negative thinking.

TREATMENT

Negative thoughts, fears, and concerns can be reduced by changing the way you think. It's like erasing an outdated hard drive on a computer that

constantly crashes and rebooting it with new, positive, inspirational information. Aim to repeat the affirmation with meaning and expectation of a positive outcome on waking and before sleep and whenever you remember during the day. Make sure you write it down, too.

Affirmations are not a cure-all, but used with flower remedies, meditation and visualization, they can be a potent mind detox tool.

MAKE THEM WORK
◆ Put passion and utter conviction into them.
◆ Express them in writing as well as verbally.
◆ Believe in them.

BREATHING

Expels toxins ◆ Replenishes the body with oxygen

Massages the internal organs ◆ Stills the mind

BREATHE OUT
Imagine you are letting go
of toxins as you exhale
stale air from your lungs.

KEY PRINCIPLES

Learning to breathe properly is an essential part of any self-healing detox program. The act of inhaling deeply to take in life-giving oxygen is believed to represent the interface between body and mind in Eastern healthcare systems such as Traditional Chinese Medicine and Ayurveda. The expansion of the diaphragm and lungs massages the internal organs and enables a greater quantity of oxygen to circulate, which allows the organs, tissues, and cells to carry out their functions efficiently.

Exhalation is a significant channel of elimination for the body and shallow breathing contributes to toxicity – if the body does not expel sufficient carbon dioxide, toxins build up. Focusing on the breath also stills an overactive mind and helps the release of toxins through visualization.

Practicing the Breath of Life exercise is the best way to relearn how to breathe and increase your oxygen intake. Wear comfortable clothing that does not restrict you.

BREATH OF LIFE

◆ Sit in a comfortable position, with your spine upright, supported by pillows if necessary. Place one hand on your abdomen and the other on your chest.
◆ Begin by taking a slow, deep breath, allowing the air to flow down to your abdomen as if inflating a balloon. Feel the hand on your abdomen rise while the hand on your chest remains still.
◆ Hold the breath for a few moments, then release it as a steady stream of air, until your abdomen and lungs are completely deflated.
◆ Repeat the inhalation, aiming to keep the hand on your chest still. Hold your breath for a few seconds then exhale, again allowing your abdomen to collapse fully to ensure that all the stale air in your body has been expelled. Try to focus solely on the breath.
◆ Try to do this for at least five minutes every day.

FLOWER REMEDIES

Help heal emotional problems ◆ Dissolve spiritual
blockages ◆ Restore harmony to body and mind

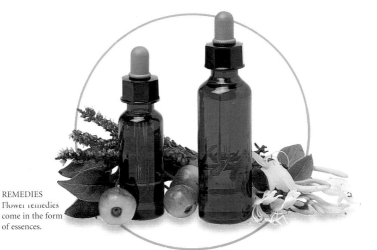

REMEDIES
Flower remedies
come in the form
of essences.

KEY PRINCIPLES

Flower essences have been used as a healing tool in many cultures for thousands of years. Practitioners believe that flowers have special properties that help heal emotional problems, thereby restoring harmony to mind and body. Flower essences work in a similar way to homeopathic remedies. Since they are a form of subtle energy, flower essences work best on the mind, emotions, and spirit.

Flower remedies can help restore the body to a state of harmony by dissolving blockages such as negative emotions. Once the body is balanced, its self-healing mechanisms can begin to function effectively.

TREATMENT

Flower essences are made by infusing individual plants and flowers in spring water. As the flowers infuse, they release their vibrational energy, which is captured in the water. The result is a tincture, which is diluted and preserved with an alcohol such as brandy or vodka. Practitioners recommend taking several drops (usually four) of the remedy daily mixed in water or dropped undiluted under the tongue. When taking more than one remedy at a time, reduce the dose to two drops of each.

Flower remedies have no side effects and are not habit-forming. They can be used safely by adults and children.

BACH FLOWER REMEDIES

Dr. Edward Bach, a London-based doctor and homeopath early in the 20th century, believed that flowers possessed properties that helped heal emotional states. Bach identified these powers intuitively by holding his hand over each flower. He devoted his life to researching flowers, isolating 38 essences with specific healing powers.

LEVEL I REMEDIES
WALNUT
Known as the link breaker, this remedy is recommended if you are undergoing major life changes. It is useful when you are starting a mind detox program since it is thought to strengthen the determination to see things through to completion and to alleviate feelings of

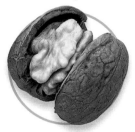

despondency and discouragement. It can help break negative cycles of behavior, such as food addictions or restrictive thought-patterns, and encourages movement toward a more positive attitude and nourishing lifestyle. Dr. Bach referred to it as "the remedy for those who have decided to take a great step forward in life, to break old conventions, to leave old limits and restrictions, and start on a new way."

HORNBEAM
This is traditionally known as the "Monday-morning feeling" remedy. It instills renewed vigour and a freshness of mind and body. Hornbeam is ideal for the level I mind detox because it

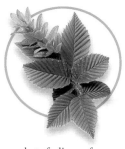

combats feelings of apathy, poor motivation, and procrastination about starting or adhering to the program.

OLIVE
Olive is a superb remedy for exhaustion and fatigue since it is said to revitalize and restore mental and physical reserves. Most people feel tired in the early stages of a detox program. Olive supports the kidney and adrenal energy, making it an ideal remedy to take during level I detox.

OAK
Like olive, oak is another restorative remedy that can provide extra energy and support when fatigue sets in. An important

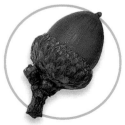

part of the level I detox program involves learning to respond to the body's signals. In the case of exhaustion, oak

essence will help you recognize that you need to allow yourself to relax and rest, instead of just continuing to battle on and deplete yourself further.

LEVEL II REMEDIES
HONEYSUCKLE
If you are nostalgic and tend to reminisce over old times, you may have become stuck in the past. The level II mind detox is concerned with letting go and moving forward emotionally. Honeysuckle is a significant remedy to take at this stage if you find yourself experiencing living-in-

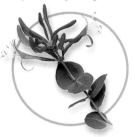

the-past patterns. This remedy helps focus your energies on the present and allows you to put the past into perspective.

WHITE CHESTNUT
If you are plagued by mental arguments and cannot let go of unhappy events, this remedy helps. When the same messages keep playing, robbing peace of mind and disturbing sleep patterns, take White Chestnut to help break obsessional thought patterns and establish constructive ways of thinking.

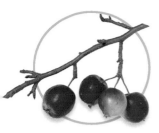

CRAB APPLE

An excellent level II detox remedy, this is a cleanser that helps purify the body. Dr. Bach described it as "the remedy which helps us to get rid of anything we do not like either in our minds or bodies." It is said to help process negative thoughts and release unresolved issues that no longer serve a useful purpose.

PINE

Long revered as a remedy of protection, Pine is thought to strengthen the spiritual defenses if your *qi* (energy) is low, leaving you more susceptible to negative energy. A key remedy for letting go of guilt, Pine is highly recommended for people who blame themselves

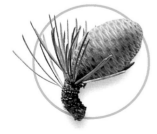

for situations that have gone wrong since it is thought to help dissolve and release remorse.

LEVEL III REMEDIES

IMPATIENS

This is the classic remedy for emotional patterns relating to the liver in Traditional Chinese Medicine (TCM): anger, a tendency to overreact, mood swings, impatience, and irritability. Impatiens releases the "pressure-cooker" feelings often experienced when the liver is in need of detoxifying – the function of the level III detox. It helps generate instead the qualities of empathy, compassion, and gentleness that, according to TCM, support the *Hun*, or spiritual soul, which resides in the liver.

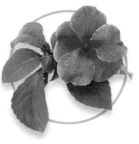

ROCK WATER

In Traditional Chinese Medicine, flexibility is a key description of the liver in harmony – an aim of the level III detox. Rock water is recommended for states of inflexibility and overrigidity, for perfectionists who constantly strive and thus are prone to becoming tense and irritable, further aggravating their liver *qi* (energy). Try it if you are so strict and inflexible that you are often in denial and never satisfied with your achievements.

HOLLY

This is an ideal remedy to take if the gallbladder is out of balance and when you experience emotions such as jealousy, envy, hatred, pent-up anger, and suppressed rage. Such emotions are likely

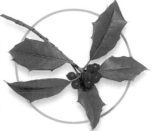

to surface when close relationships come to an end. The body cannot detoxify on an emotional level when these feelings are held fast within. The Holly remedy can transmute bitter emotions into their opposites – compassion and love.

SCLERANTHUS

Take this remedy when you experience mental indecision, changeable moods, and fluctuating symptoms, all of which, in Traditional Chinese Medicine, point to an imbalance of the liver. Scleranthus enhances the level III mind detox by helping improve clarity of the mind. This effect enables you to feel more organized and confident about your ability to take a precise plan of action.

SPIRIT DETOX

"THE GREAT MALADY OF THE TWENTIETH
CENTURY ... IS LOSS OF SOUL. WHEN THE SOUL
IS NEGLECTED, IT DOESN'T JUST GO AWAY; IT
APPEARS IN OBSESSIONS, ADDICTIONS,
VIOLENCE, AND LOSS OF MEANING. IF THE
SOUL'S CAPACITY FOR CREATIVITY IS NOT
HONORED IT WILL WREAK HAVOC."

THOMAS MOORE

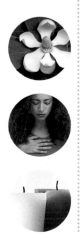

THE IMPORTANCE OF THE SOUL

Nourishment of the soul is the foundation of life and living. The trials of daily life that consume so much energy can prevent us from focusing on much deeper issues. We need to take a comprehensive look at the health of the soul.

ANALYZING THE SOUL

Using detox to attain peace of mind involves taking an introspective and comprehensive look at the health and balance of body, mind, and soul. But there is a problem with analyzing the soul. The dictionary's definition, "spirit or immaterial part of man, the seat of human personality, intellect, will, and emotions," is much too general to be of use. We each have our own unique, deeply personal idea of what "soul" means.

Many of the ancient healing traditions, with their far-reaching wisdom and remarkable insight, respected the body as a whole. Healing the body also involved healing the highest level – the soul. The main objective was to protect the soul while weaknesses in the body and mind were treated.

Today, modern science (backed by the World Health Organization) accepts the validity of the concept of a biological energy that radiates outward from a living body. This biological energy creates an electrical field, known as an aura, which surrounds us; it can even be measured and photographed electronically. The level II mind detox program includes a meditation created to protect and reinforce this phenomenon.

MAKING TIME FOR THE SOUL

Many people are aware of the importance of "soul-time" – time to be alone, to reflect and be still – but all too often, it is a casualty of a busy schedule. Although the storms of life can throw us out of balance, simply being aware of the constant fluctuation between being centered and at peace or off-center and in a state of turmoil can be useful. It can make us more aware of the here and now and encourage us to make a positive effort to retain our inner centre and equilibrium.

The spiritual detox programs in this book are designed to help you find time for your soul. Without spending time alone to appreciate and enjoy solitude, to think, dream, feel, develop, and be still, you cannot grow and evolve spiritually. But once you begin to enjoy this time to reflect, meditate, and be creative, you will find yourself reserving time to take these vital steps to a lifelong journey of nourishing the soul.

MAKING AND USING A SACRED SPACE

Creating a sacred space in your home sets up the right atmosphere to develop this process. To make this space a tranquil haven of peace and a special place for you to be alone, you should:

• play music that touches your soul
• burn aromatherapy oils that instill a sense of well-being
• let the soft glow of candles light your sacred place.

During meditation and visualization, use your energy to evoke vibrant images of yourself feeling strong and radiantly healthy. Add to this a desire to awaken your body's natural healing mechanisms to encourage them to overcome any imbalances. For major changes on a spiritual level to be possible, you must lay a firm foundation on which to build. This means first ensuring that your body is physically nourished with proper food, regular exercise, and sufficient rest.

The holistic approach to detox is vital. Your focus is not just on your spirit, nor just on your body, but on your entire physical, spiritual and emotional being. Before you begin to meditate it is essential that you are properly grounded in your body. The deeper your roots reach into your core, the steadier your foundations will be and the higher your soul will soar.

Affirmation

"Today I will lovingly nurture the divinity that resides in my soul."

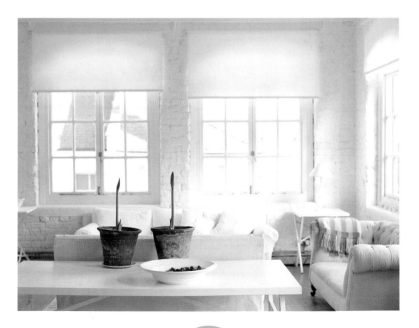

PROGRAM FOR LEVEL I

This first level is concerned with visualizing your body without problems and sensing it radiating health and vitality. It is also about feeling safe and secure and allowing any worries to melt away.

CLEANSING PREPARATION

You should do this meditation before any of the others. Grounding activities include any work with the earth such as gardening or walking in the countryside.

Grounding Meditation

◆ Begin by finding a peaceful place to relax (*see page 107*). Close your eyes, begin to deepen your breathing and gently let any thoughts float by like clouds in the sky. Now imagine that with your next exhalation, a root grows from the base of your spine and smaller roots spread from the end of your toes and travel deep into the center of the earth.

◆ As you inhale, feel your body absorbing energy from Mother Earth; visualize this energy as a golden liquid that fills your entire body. Now feel it turning darker as it absorbs all your negative energy. As you exhale, feel this liquid drain down from the top of your head, taking with it all stress and worry.

◆ With your next breath, visualize golden waves of energy flowing up and feel it washing over you. As you exhale, sense a beam of clear white light entering through the point at the top of your head. Feel this light permeate and cleanse body and soul on an even deeper level.

◆ Repeat several times this cycle of inhaling the golden liquid from the earth and exhaling and drawing down the white healing light from the heavens. Sense your energy becoming stronger and begin to move your fingers and toes, feeling yourself revitalized and grounded.

◆ Continue with the next meditation, or the ones for levels II or III.

Meditation for Nurturing and Finding the Light Within

♦ Prepare to meditate (*see page 114*).

♦ Feel the warmth and energy of the golden color that resonates with the Earth element. Visualize a golden liquid traveling through your digestive tract, strengthening and supporting the stomach and spleen.

♦ Take your focus to the left side of your body near the ribs where your spleen and stomach are located; take a moment to honor these organs and their functions. Let the healing light flow into these organs, so strengthening their ability to receive and transform Mother Earth's produce into vital energy for you.

♦ If you feel bloated, carry extra weight or fluid, or suffer from digestive problems, low energy, or food allergies, then feel this light energize and give you the power to clear any blockages and shed light on any unresolved emotional issues connected to nourishment, nurturing, and low self-esteem.

♦ Go deeper and see if you can sense the origins of these feelings of insecurity and worry. Now wrap these emotions and events in a golden web of light and watch as the golden threads dissolve these feelings until there is nothing remaining but golden glitter.

♦ Reflect on your relationship with food and make a commitment to become more consciously aware of what encourages you to use food as a crutch. See yourself being guided to eat more wholesome, nourishing foods that really make you feel vibrant and alive.

♦ Develop an inner knowing that you are special; feel love for yourself. Believe in yourself and your self-worth and constantly feed yourself with loving and constructive affirmations. Respect your body, your uniqueness, and your gifts.

♦ Feel waves of golden energy washing over your whole body, filling your mind, body, and spirit with a deep sense of satisfaction and fulfillment. Sense your energy becoming stronger and begin to move your fingers and toes, feeling yourself revitalized and grounded.

♦ In your own time, open your eyes and stretch your body out.

Your Ideal Picture

Visualize your body without any problems, radiating health and vitality. Imagine yourself as the "ideal you." Expand that picture – believe it, feel it, and see yourself exuding confidence, energy, happiness, and health. Now think of a tremendously happy time in your life. Recall the feelings of love, joy, and confidence that you experienced at that time and feel them flooding your body.

PROGRAM FOR LEVEL II

This level II spirit-detoxing program aims to cleanse and reinforce the emotions and spirit – our protective sphere – so that the immune system is also protected and the lungs are strengthened.

PROTECTING THE SPIRIT

The protective meditation is for when you feel drained after interacting with negative people or situations, and it is an invaluable tool that helps cleanse the mind and spirit and regenerate energy.

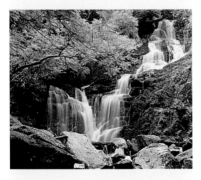

Before doing the level II meditations you need to deepen your breathing and relax your body. Do the Breath of Life (*see page 100*) and the grounding meditation (*see page 108*).

Protective Meditation

◆ To cleanse your body of any negative feelings, imagine that you are standing under a waterfall of crystal light. Feel this light wash over your body, sweeping with it any negative energies. See the brilliant light flowing around your aura and clearing any darkness, allowing your energy field to be refreshed and full of light. Allow the crystal-clear energy to permeate your physical body, filling it with luminous light. Imagine the negativity flowing down out of your body and into the earth. Give thanks that the negativity has been released and to the earth for transmuting it.

◆ Now surround yourself in a golden protective mist. Intensify this mist around the back of your body and head because this is where you are most vulnerable and need the greatest amount of protection. Then see the outer edges of the mist clearly forming a golden sphere of protection around your being that allows healing energy in but prevents negative vibrations from entering your space.

◆ Reinforce the golden sphere of protection through the day to keep your defenses strong.

Letting Go Meditation

◆ Imagine yourself seated beneath a tree in the autumn. Focus on a branch of the tree with a leaf about to fall. As you watch this leaf fall gently to the earth, imagine that it represents a feeling, a situation or a relationship that no longer has relevance in your life. Let it go and be one with the cycle of nature – it is the time to release, to let go of emotions and events that do not sustain you. Don't be frightened of experiencing loss – it is a necessary part of life's cycle, so feel any grief as you release this memory.

◆ Repeat this process attaching old hurts and labels that people have put upon you. Fully experience the emotion as you watch each leaf on its journey from the tree to the ground; look at the pile of leaves on the earth and give thanks that you have been able to let go of these memories. Reflect on the deeper meaning of the difficulties you have experienced; view them as challenges that tested your soul and helped you grow spiritually.

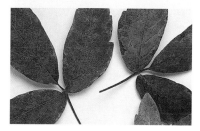

◆ Now visualize a clear, white healing light entering the top of your head and feel it cleanse your mind, bringing with it a sense of peace and calm. See this white light flow down your body into your lungs and allow your breath to deepen. Breathe in the light and exhale with a large sigh, releasing any remaining stress held in your body and ensuring that stale air is properly expelled. Let the out breath dissolve and remove any remaining feelings of grief; allow the clean air you inhale to cleanse and heal.

◆ See this brilliant light flowing around your entire body, cleansing and strengthening your lymphatic system. Take another deep breath through your nose, allowing the white light to travel down to your gut; intensify the light and feel it clearing your body of all the mental and physical toxins stored in your intestines. With your breathing becoming deeper with every inhalation, visualize the good bacteria growing and any parasites, *Candida*, viruses, or other bacteria losing their power. See them being dissolved and destroyed by the powerful white healing light and imagine that any toxins are eliminated. Visualize clearly now your body bathed in this white light: you feel cleansed, powerful, regenerated, and at peace.

◆ Now, take a slow, deep breath and release; open your eyes and take a big stretch.

PROGRAM FOR LEVEL III

This third-level program focuses on the spiritual detoxification of the liver and gallbladder, releasing negative emotions such as anger and resentment, and helping you plan ahead for a new future.

DETOXIFYING DEEP-SEATED EMOTIONS

Prepare yourself carefully prior to beginning this meditation (*see pages 108 and 114*).

Dissolving anger

◆ Visualize yourself sitting beneath the boughs of a mighty oak tree in a woodland glade in spring. Become aware of the new growth and of leaf buds bursting open on slender young saplings that gently sway in the spring breeze. In Traditional Chinese Medicine a healthy liver is compared to a young tree that is flexible yet firmly rooted into the earth, its movements graceful and fluid.

◆ Imagine your feet on a velvet green carpet of new grass beneath you; absorb the rich green color and allow this to flow up your body. Feel it intensify around your neck and shoulder area and sense it melting and releasing any tension held in these muscles.

◆ Feeling lighter and freer, let the green glow travel to the right side of your ribcage where your liver and gallbladder are located. Increase the fresh spring color around these two organs, letting it seep into them; intensify the energy and feel it giving strength and enabling them to detoxify your body and mind more efficiently of negative emotions and physical toxins. The liver is the seat of anger, the area where irritation, frustration, and even rage can reside; begin to sense if you have any anger held within or any unresolved grudges or resentment, perhaps from a time when you were unable to express these emotions?

◆ Allow a soft green mist to envelope both your gallbladder and liver and feel this dissolving any negativity, rage, anger, or hatred. Can you find forgiveness in your heart and give yourself permission to release this unresolved anger? It eats away inside of you creating hurt and resentment, depleting and congesting your *qi*. Feel these toxic emotions melting and reducing in both size and importance until finally they evaporate and disappear in the mist.

♦ Take a few moments to finally reflect on this release and feel a sense of peace left behind from the cooling and refreshing mist.

♦ Now feel your body energized and clear. Send energy now to your kidneys, located around the back of your waist, and see them becoming stronger and producing an abundance of vital energy, which, in turn, benefits your entire body.

You may need to repeat this meditation several times to truly let go of some anger but know that you will process this in your own time.

Making a Fresh Start

♦ Now the liver is clearer, it is time to sow your dreams, plans, and aspirations. Feel the surge of this spring energy inspiring and encouraging you to make a fresh start and to plan ahead for a new future, make a commitment to become more organized, to have a true sense of purpose and direction, and to make your life plan a reality. Start to visualize some of the things that you really would like to manifest in your life.

♦ Paint a picture in your imagination where you see these dreams very clearly and you are the focal point of your dream. Build the dream and create the

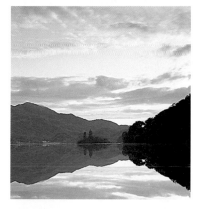

reality. Create these vivid and real pictures and feelings in your subconscious; intensify your desire and belief that these dreams will one day come into manifestation.

♦ Look forward to this time in this meditation as your time to put out into the Universe the vision that will help you create positive changes in your life. Fill your body with light and hope of a brighter future where new doors will open. Allow peace and tranquility to envelop your mind, body, and spirit. Feel your energy becoming stronger and move your fingers and toes; take a deep breath and sense new life and vitality enter your body.

♦ Open your eyes and stretch your body.

MEDITATION & VISUALIZATION

Promote a deep sense of tranquility ◆ Reduce stress

levels ◆ Stimulate the body's self-healing powers

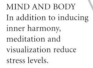

MIND AND BODY
In addition to inducing inner harmony, meditation and visualization reduce stress levels.

KEY PRINCIPLES

Long recognized by all major religions and healthcare systems, East and West, as vital for well-being, meditation allows you to access a spiritual state beyond everyday consciousness.

Psychologically, it promotes a deep sense of tranquility and helps you achieve and maintain serenity and equilibrium. Physiologically, it has been shown to lower blood pressure and reduce stress and anxiety levels, thus helping the brain function smoothly.

Visualization also uses the power of the mind to heal by creating positive mental images that guide and stimulate the body's natural healing abilities.

HOW THEY WORK

Recent research into the body/mind link confirms the power of these two therapies to reduce stress levels. This is important in detoxing: high levels of the stress hormones epinephrine and cortisol stimulate enzymes in the liver and kidneys that can activate harmful detoxification pathways.

Thoughts may seem intangible, but are capable of producing changes in the physical body. Using visualization helps you access your subconscious mind and evoke positive physical and psychological responses. This helps to reduce stress levels, a key aim of the detox plan.

BASIC MEDITATION

◆ Sit up in a comfortable, supported position.

◆ Close your eyes, focusing on exhaling stale air and inhaling pure, fresh air.

◆ Remain focused on the breath. When thoughts arise, acknowledge them and return to your focus.

◆ Continue for as long as is comfortable – a few minutes at first, building up to 20 minutes a day.

◆ To conclude, open your eyes and try to retain a sense of inner peace.

EXERCISE

Improves the flow of life energy ◆ Balances the body, mind, and spirit ◆ Enhances the immune system

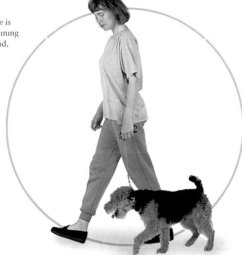

STAYING ACTIVE
Regular mild exercise is invaluable in maintaining balance in body, mind, and spirit.

KEY PRINCIPLES

The Chinese approach to exercise is very different from that of the West. In Traditional Chinese Medicine (TCM), exercise techniques such as t'ai chi are considered to be invaluable for maintaining balance and preventing illness, but strenuous exercise is not endorsed, especially in cold seasons, as it is thought to deplete vital *qi* (energy). Only gentle forms of exercise, such as swimming or walking, which promote the circulation of blood and *qi* throughout the body, are recommended.

HOW IT WORKS

Doctors of TCM believe that not exercising contributes to stagnation and congestion in the body and may lead to the development of illness. Stretching is thought to improve the flow of *qi* in the meridians (energy pathways), having a beneficial impact on the organs. For this reason, stretches designed to increase flexibility and to support the relevant body systems are recommended for each level of the program (*see page 117*).

It is important to listen to your body; doing levels II and III, you may feel fit enough to combine more active regimes with the restorative programs set out on page 116, but do not push yourself. If you have a medical condition, always check with your doctor first.

● **CAUTION**
Strenuous exercise can decrease immunity for six hours and increase antioxidant requirements.

EXERCISE & DETOX
Detoxing at all levels is helped by exercise.
◆ At level I, gentle exercise can build up your strength. Rest is equally important if you feel fatigued.
◆ At level II, moderate cardiovascular activity can increase oxygen uptake, improving your immune system.
◆ At level III, deepening stretches and using more dynamic forms of movement, such as yoga, may dissipate liver stagnation.

LEVEL I EXERCISE

Some form of movement is essential at level I, but if you are excluding certain foods from your diet, you may lack the energy for a great deal. Try gentle exercise, such as walking, for 15–20 minutes, 3–5 times a week, followed by the Earth element stretch (*see opposite*). Follow an exercise regimen you enjoy – swimming, gentle

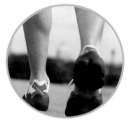

cycling, country walks – the aim at level I is to inspire you to take up a new way of life that will continue long after you finish the detox program.

As your body gets stronger and your energy levels improve, increase the duration and intensity of the exercise, but always be aware of how your body feels during and after a workout. If you feel exhaustion that lasts into the next day, reduce the program and get more rest until your vitality increases: rest and relaxation are highly restorative. At level I you are aiming to rebuild and restore your energy levels, so listen to your body. The Earth element stretch enhances the spleen and nourishes the "Mental" soul (*Yi*).

LEVEL II EXERCISE

In Traditional Chinese Medicine, the supreme function of the lungs is to receive energy, bringing energy into the body. Breathing, like eating, is considered a fundamental way to replenish energy levels.

Regular cardiovascular exercise makes breathing deeper and more frequent, increasing oxygen uptake in the body and exercising the lung muscles. Aerobic exercise also enhances detox work on poor circulation or a

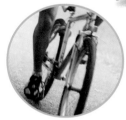

sluggish lymphatic system. Swimming is one of the best forms of exercise for stimulating lymphatic system drainage.

At level II you should increase your exercise sessions to 30–45 minutes, five times a week, to gain maximum cardiovascular and respiratory benefit. Cycling, power-walking, gentle jogging, tennis, swimming, and aerobics are all suitable – just make sure it is something you can maintain. Follow each session with the Earth and Metal element exercises (*see opposite*). The Metal element exercise lifts the "Bodily" soul (*P'o*) and *wei qi*.

LEVEL III EXERCISE

Movement, flexibility, and flow are all paramount at level III. Continue with moderate cardiovascular exercise as suggested at level II and, when it feels right, introduce more challenging forms of exercise, such as yoga, to encourage the flow of *qi*

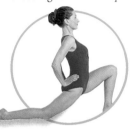

(energy) and blood in the body, supplying more oxygen to the tissues.

The liver plays a vital role in filtering blood and directing it to nourish the muscles during exercise. If its function of cleansing and renewing the blood is impaired, this can cause stiffness. In Traditional Chinese Medicine (TCM), the Wood element controls ligaments and tendons and their inter-action with muscles. TCM views excessive exercise and too many late nights as depleting blood and *qi*, so go to bed before 11pm if you feel stiff and tired.

Include in your exercise plan the Wood element stretch (*opposite*), and the Earth and Metal element exercises, too. The Wood element stretch encourages grace and harmonizes the "Spiritual" soul (*Hun*).

LEVEL I: STRETCH TO ENHANCE DIGESTION AND SUPPORT THE EARTH ELEMENT

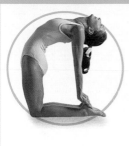

In a kneeling position, place your hands on your hips for support. Slowly inhale, lengthening your spine. Exhale, pushing your hips forwards. Gently curve your spine backward, drop your head back and, if you feel strong enough, let your hands drop to your heels. If you prefer, at first, simply keep your hands on your hips to support the lower back. Breathe, relax, and feel the stretch down the front of your thighs and torso. Hold for 10–30 seconds, then gently come back to a kneeling position and curl forward in a ball, allowing your head to rest on the floor. Relax, breathing deeply, and repeat. It may take weeks to achieve a deeper stretch, so be patient!

LEVEL II: EXERCISE TO ENHANCE BREATHING AND SUPPORT THE METAL ELEMENT

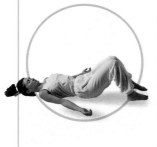

Practice this exercise in a peaceful environment. Lie on your back with knees bent and feet hip-width apart, firmly on the floor. Allow your arms to flop out at your sides with the palms facing upward. Keep the back of your neck gently extended and your shoulders relaxed. Close your eyes. As you begin to deepen your breathing, allow any tension in your shoulders to melt away and let your mind release any mental stress you are carrying. Continue to breathe deeply in this position by practicing the Breath of Life exercise (see page 100). When you feel ready, bring your knees to your chest and gently hug them: this brings relief to the lower back and is a very comfortable position to rest in.

LEVEL III: STRETCH TO GIVE BALANCE AND TO SUPPORT THE WOOD ELEMENT

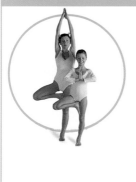

This yoga pose may not be as physically demanding as many postures, but its challenge lies in its need for mental focus. Take up a standing position and place your weight on to your right foot. Take your left foot with your right hand and place it on the inside of your right thigh. Now fix your gaze on a point in front of you to help you balance, and bring both hands together at your chest in a prayer position. If you feel steady, lift your arms upward, bring your hands together and stretch your fingers toward the heavens. Breathe gently and try to hold the position for 30 seconds before releasing your foot to the ground. Repeat on the other leg.

DAILY DETOX PROGRAM FOR LIFE

This detox program is not daunting and will fit easily into your daily life. You can follow it every day or incorporate it once a week into your routine, using it along with or independently of the main programs in the book.

Starting the Day

On waking, remind yourself of why you want to detox with the affirmation below.

BREATHING EXERCISE
Practice the Breath of Life exercise (*see page 100*). This focus on breathing is designed to expel up to three-quarters of the waste accumulated overnight by the body.

ENERGY EXERCISE
Warm up, then do the stretches suggested for your detox level (*see page 117*) to encourage the proper flow of *qi* (energy).

Affirmation
I make a commitment to respect, nurture, and care for my body, my temple. It is safe to let go of anything that does not nourish my mind, my body, and my spirit.

If you are new to detoxing, take it slowly: enjoy the changes it will bring, add healing therapies (*see pages 26–33*) to your daily regime and appreciate the fresh, natural, organic foods, herbs, and spices you are eating.

During the Day

BREAKFAST
Choose from the breakfast menu selection (*see page 38*), ensuring

Skin Brush and Shower
◆ Do the skin-brushing routine for 2–3 minutes (*see page 81*).
◆ Take a warm shower, then switch to cold water for half a minute to encourage blood flow and lymph movement.
◆ Apply a natural moisturizer or light oil such as jojoba oil to your skin.

a good mix of the fruits and cereals appropriate for your detox level. Accompany with ginger tea (*see page 71*), green tea, or a fresh vegetable juice.

DRINKS FOR THE DAY
Drink a glass of water hourly to help flush out toxins. Also drink herbal teas and fresh juices.

MIDMORNING SNACK

Select from the following: organic vegetable juice; natural live sheep or goat's yogurt; a handful of mixed nuts and seeds; rice or oatcakes with a nut butter spread.

LUNCH

Choose from the lunch menu selection (*see page 39*).

MIDDAY EXERCISE

Have a brisk walk or a swim on your lunch hour, especially if you didn't have time to do the energy exercise at the start of the day. This helps the body eliminate toxins and stimulates the circulatory and lymphatic systems. Close with the stretches for the start of the day (*see opposite*).

MIDAFTERNOON SNACK

Select another option from the snacks suggested for midmorning (*see above*), which are also ideal for this time of day.

In the Evening

MINISPIRITUAL CLEANSE

Once home, release the stresses and strains of the day by doing the Simple Cleansing Grounding Meditation (*see page 108*).

EVENING MEAL

Be creative, adding lots of fresh herbs and spices to your cooking, and enjoy making and eating your evening meal (*see New Eating Habits, page 91*).

Spa Treatment

- Run a bath, adding Dead Sea salts or a few drops of an essential oil (*see page 29*).
- Lie back and massage the reflex and acupressure points for your detox level while soaking (*see pages 80–5*).
- Focus on the affirmations for your detox level (*see page 99*).
- Practice the Breath of Life exercise (*see page 100*).
- Pull the plug, but remain in the bath. Imagine the day's stresses and toxins draining away with the bathwater.

EVENING DRINKS

To stimulate the digestion, make a cup of ginger tea (*see page 71*). For a good night's sleep, choose a cup of chamomile tea.

BEFORE BED

This is the ideal time to meditate (*see page 114*); focusing on mind and spirit ensures that you are grounded and peaceful.

SLEEP

Be sure to get eight hours' sleep. This allows the physical and mental systems to rest, repair, and regenerate themselves.

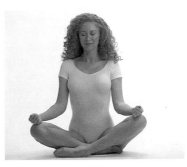

GLOSSARY

ACUTE DISEASE Disorder or symptom that comes on suddenly and is usually of short duration. Symptoms may be severe, such as high fever or severe pain.

ANTIOXIDANTS Substances that counteract the harmful properties of free radicals found in the environment.

BACTERIA Single-cell microorganisms, commonly called "germs," that exist in air, soil, and water. Some bacteria, such as the acidophilus found in natural yogurt, have a beneficial effect on health. Others can be harmful and cause infections.

BIOFLAVONOIDS Natural antioxidants found in valuable quantities in some fruits, such as berries, and in vegetables such as sweet peppers.

CHRONIC DISEASE Disorder or set of symptoms that persist for a long time; may show little change from day to day.

ESSENTIAL FATTY ACIDS Unsaturated fats that are essential for health. The body cannot make certain essential polyunsaturated fats and these must be gained from food. Omega-3 fats (alpha-linoleic acid) are found in oily fish and linseed; omega-6 fats (linoleic acid) are in nuts and seeds.

FREE RADICALS Reactive and unstable substances that are continually being made and broken down in the body. They have the potential to damage cells, causing cell degeneration.

FUNCTIONAL MEDICINE A healthcare system in which the emphasis is on optimizing organ and body system function.

IMMUNOGLOBULIN G (IgG) The major immunoglobulins (a type of protein, also called an antibody) in the blood. They play a central role in allergic reactions, binding onto antigens in the cells of the immune system, destroying the microorganisms that carry them.

IMMUNE SYSTEM A collection of cells and proteins that enable the body to recognize and identify foreign invaders such as bacteria and viruses, and to neutralize or eliminate them.

LEAKY GUT SYNDROME A condition in which the intestinal wall is damaged, allowing both normal and toxic residue to leak into the body.

METABOLISM Collective term for all the chemical processes in the body that break down or build up ingested substances for optimum utilization.

PECTIN A soluble fiber found in fruit that enhances the body's ability to prevent absorption of toxic compounds and reduces bowel transit time.

PHASE I DETOXIFICATION A liver detoxification pathway where some toxins are neutralized to be processed by phase II enzymes. This process often creates more toxic compounds which are also sent to phase II for detoxifying.

PHASE II DETOXIFICATION A liver detoxification pathway that uses conjugation, a process whereby small chemicals are attached to a toxin, either neutralizing it or making it more easy to eliminate, through urine or bile.

PHYTOCHEMICALS Also called phytonutrients, these are chemical constituents found in plants which have a positive effect on health and well-being.

PHYTOESTROGENS Plant hormones or substances found in some plants and foods that mimic estrogen hormones (essential for the healthy functioning of the reproductive system).

PROANTHROCYANIDINS Antioxidant flavonoids that give rise to the blue/red pigments found in fruits such as berries.

STANDARDIZED EXTRACT A precise measure of an herb, ensuring that it contains the exact concentration of the active ingredient in the plant.

TOXINS Poisonous compounds produced by disease-causing bacteria in the environment, plants, and animals. They may be breathed in, ingested, or enter the body via cuts and wounds.

TRANS FATS Saturated fats made when oils are hydrogenated to harden them for use in margarine and processed foods.

VIRUSES The smallest known types of infective agent. Viral infections can be trivial or very serious.

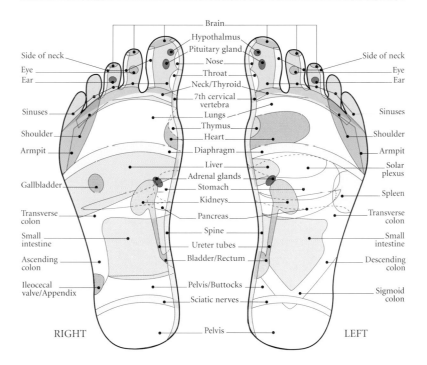

RIGHT　　LEFT

REFLEXOLOGY

Practitioners of reflexology believe that this therapy can stimulate the body's natural healing powers. These maps of the soles and sides of the feet show the precise areas, or reflex points, corresponding to areas of the body, which reflexologists massage. Reflexology therapy is explained on page 30.

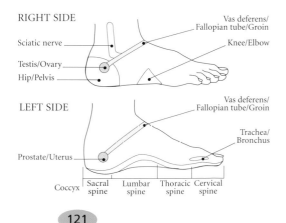

BIBLIOGRAPHY

The following is a selected list of further material that you may find useful.

Bateson-Koch, Carolee
Allergies: Disease in Disguise
(Alive Books, 1998)

Bayly, Doreen E.
Reflexology Today: the Stimulation of the Body's Healing Forces through Foot Massage
(Healing Arts Press, 1982)

Brewer, Sarah
Candida Albicans
(Thorsons, 1997)

Chaitow, Leon
The Antibiotic Crisis: Antibiotic Alternatives
(Thorsons, 1998)

Chopra, Deepak
The Seven Spiritual Laws of Success
(Bantam Press, 1996)

Clark, Susan
The Sunday Times Vitality Cookbook
(HarperCollins, 1999)

D'Adamo, Peter J. and Whitney, Catherine
Eat Right for Your Type
(Putnam, 1997)

Davis, Patricia
Aromatherapy: an A–Z
(C. W. Daniel, 1995)

Erasmus, Udo
Fats that Heal, Fats that Kill
(Alive Books, 1999)

Grant, Doris and Joice, Jean
Food Combining for Health
(Thorsons, 1991)

Gursche, Siegfried and Zoltan, Rona
Encyclopedia of Natural Healing
(Alive Books, 1998)

Gursche, Siegfried
Healing with Herbal Juices
(Alive Books, 1993)

Harper, Jennifer
Nine Ways to Body Wisdom, Blending Natural Therapies to Nourish Body, Emotions and Soul
(Thorsons, 2000)

Kaptchuk, Ted J.
Chinese Medicine: the Web That Has No Weaver
(Century, 1987)

Marsden, Kathryn
The Food Combining Diet: Lose Weight and Stay Healthy with the Hay System
(Thorsons, 1993)

McTaggart, Lynne
What Doctors Don't Tell You
(Thorsons, 1996)

Mills, Simon
The Complete Guide to Modern Herbalism
(Thorsons, 1994)

Mojay, Gabriel
Aromatherapy for Healing the Spirit
(Gaia Books, 1996)

Myss, Caroline
Why People Don't Heal and How They Can
(Bantam Press, 1998)

Pizzorno, Joseph
Total Wellness
(Prima Health, 1998)

Rechelbacher, Horst
Aveda Rituals
(Ebury Press, 1999)

Scheffer, Mechthild
Bach Flower Therapy: Theory and Practice
(Thorsons, 1986)

Sellar, Wanda
The Directory of Essential Oils (C. W. Daniel, 1992)

Van Straten, Michael
Healing Foods
(The Ivy Press, 1997)

Vogel, H. C. A.
Nature Doctor: Manual of Traditional Medicine
(Mainstream Publishing Company, 1990)

Young, Jacqueline
Acupressure Step by Step
(Thorsons, 1998)

Young, Jacqueline
Acupressure for Health: a Complete Self-care Manual
(Thorsons, 1994)

The Green Guide
(Green Guide Publishing)
An annually published eco-directory available from:
020 7354 2709
www.greenguideonline.com

MEDITATION MATERIAL

Harper, Jennifer
Seasons of the Soul
A guided meditation CD written and recorded by Jennifer Harper; includes extended versions of all the meditations used in this book together with other healing exercises. Available from Aveda stores or by mail order from:
08450 606070 (UK)
0044 113 388 5230
 (non-UK)
www.jenniferharper.com

USEFUL ADDRESSES

ORGANIZATIONS

American Academy of Medical Acupuncture
4929 Wilshire Boulevard
Los Angeles, CA 90010
(323) 937–5514
www.medicalacupuncture.org

The American Association of Naturopathic Physicians
8201 Greensboro Drive
McLean, VA 22102
(877) 969–2267
www.naturopathic.org

American Dietetic Association
216 W Jackson Boulevard
Chicago, IL 60606
(800) 877–1600
www.eatright.org

Friends of the Earth
1025 Vermont Ave. NW
Washington, DC 20005–6303
(202) 783–7400
www.foe.org

Greenpeace USA
702 H Street NW
Washington, DC 20001
(800) 326–0959
www.greenpeace.org

Jennifer Harper
PO Box 150, Woking
Surrey GU23 6XS
www.jenniferharper.com

National Center for Complementary and Alternative Medicine
PO Box 7923
Gaithersburg, MD 20898
(888) 644–6226
nccam.nih.gov

National Association for Holistic Aromatherapy
4509 Interlake Avenue N
Seattle, WA 98103–6773
(888) 275–6242
www.naha.org

National Federation of Spiritual Healers
Healer referral line:
011–44–891 616080
Heart Awakening Project Inc.
PO Box 4195
Cave Creek, AS 85327
www.heartawakening.com

American Herbalists Guild
1931 Gaddis Road
Canton, GA 30115
(770) 751–6021
www.americanherbalistsguild.com

PRODUCT SUPPLIERS

Aveda Inc.
4000 Pheasant Ridge Drive
MN 55449–7106
(612) 783–4000
www.aveda.com
Organic, environmentally friendly personal products.

Collega
1800 Birchmount Road
Toronto, Ontario M1P 2H7
(416) 754–1444
Canadian distributor of Aveda products.

Klamath Blue Green Algae
PO Box 1626
Mount Shasta, CA 96097
(800) 327–1956
www.klamathbluegreen.com

Oasis Esthetique
1231 St. Catherine Street W
Montreal, Quebec H3G 1P5
(514) 286–9146
www.drhauschka.com
Canadian distributor of Dr. Hauschka skincare products.

Origins
6200 Commerce Center Drive
Groveport, OH 43125
(800) 674–4467
www.origins.com

Solgar Vitamin and Herb Company, Inc.
500 Willow Tree Road
Leonia, NJ 07605
(877) 765–4274
www.solgar.com

The Wild Herb and Spice Company
PO Box 4885
Buffalo Grove, IL 60089
(800) 243–5242

Udo's Choice Oil (flax oil)
Flora Inc.
805 East Badger Road
Lynden, WA 98264
(360) 454–2110
www.savant-health.com
Essential fatty acid flax seed oils.

ORGANIC FOOD SUPPLIERS

American Health & Nutrition, Inc.
3990 Varsity Drive
Ann Arbor, MI 48108
(734) 677–5570
www.organictrading.com
Nationwide mail-order service for organic fresh produce.

Beta Pure Foods
Morr Pure Foods, Inc.
335 Spreckels Drive
Aptos, CA 95003
(831) 685–6565
www.betapure.com

Hill Foods Ltd.
#109–3650 Bonneville Place
Burnaby, BC V3N 4T7
(604) 421–3100
www.hillsfoods.com
Mail-order naturally produced meat reared at the farm.

INDEX

Page numbers in **bold** indicate main entries for foods and supplements. These include full details of nutrient and phytochemical content, detox and health benefits, naturopathic and Traditional Chinese Medicine properties, and recommended intake. These details have not normally been indexed separately.

ACKNOWLEDGMENTS

AUTHOR'S ACKNOWLEDGMENTS

I would like to sincerely thank my associate and dear friend Kim Knight for her incredible support and guidance. Her encouragement, belief, and love goes beyond what mere words can convey. The same is true of my dearest mother Mary, for this and for her devotion and understanding. I would like to honor and thank an exceptional soul who has graced my life, giving unconditional love, support, friendship, and laughter – life without your special presence, Torquil, would never be the same again. Thanks to Keith Harding of Goodness Gracious for my portrait photograph, and Dana, my trusted and loyal "house angel." Finally, I would like to acknowledge the expertise of two leading nutritionists, Mike Curly, biochemist and international lecturer, and author Stephen Terrass for their technical input and scientific backup. Thank you both for your genuine interest in the work I do and in this specific project.

PUBLISHER'S ACKNOWLEDGMENTS

The publishers would like to thank the editors of Natural Health® magazine for their review, Sue Bosanko for the index, and Carla Masson for editorial assistance. The publishers would also like to thank the following for their kind permission to reproduce their photographs: Joe Cornish (110, 113); Alistair Hughes (119); Sandra Lousada (31, 34 bottom, 80 bottom right, 84, 86 middle); David Murray and Jules Selmes (27 left, 86 bottom); Stephen Oliver (33); Guy Ryecart (1 center, 28, 75 right, 99, 102 top, 103 bottom left, 104 bottom).